COVID-19: Origin, Impact and Management (Part 2)

Edited by

Tahmeena Khan
Department of Chemistry
Integral University, Lucknow
India

&

Alfred J. Lawrence
Department of Chemistry
Isabella Thoburn College, Lucknow
India

COVID-19: Origin, Impact and Management (Part 2)

Editors: Tahmeena Khan & Alfred J. Lawrence

ISBN (Online): 978-981-5165-94-4

ISBN (Print): 978-981-5165-95-1

ISBN (Paperback): 978-981-5165-96-8

First published in 2023.

need for a court order if at any point you breach any terms of this License Agreement. In no event will any delay or failure by Bentham Science Publishers in enforcing your compliance with this License Agreement constitute a waiver of any of its rights.

3. You acknowledge that you have read this License Agreement, and agree to be bound by its terms and conditions. To the extent that any other terms and conditions presented on any website of Bentham Science Publishers conflict with, or are inconsistent with, the terms and conditions set out in this License Agreement, you acknowledge that the terms and conditions set out in this License Agreement shall prevail.

Bentham Science Publishers Pte. Ltd.
80 Robinson Road #02-00
Singapore 068898
Singapore
Email: subscriptions@benthamscience.net

BENTHAM
SCIENCE

CONTENTS

FOREWORD I

I feel it a pleasure to write forward to the book titled "COVID-19: Origin, Impact and Management" edited by Dr. Alfred Lawrence and Dr. Tahmeena Khan. The SARS-CoV-2 or COVID-19 pandemic has jolted the entire world at different levels. It is not only the health sector that has been greatly impacted, but human life has suffered at multi-levels, be it psychological well-being, economic upheaval or discrimination in caregiving at home as faced by women. The education sector also saw reform as online mode took over. The situation is more severe and grim in developing countries and it is very important to find out the vulnerable groups, having access to lesser means of protection and prevention.

This innovative book is an interesting reading material as the assorted chapters cater to different aspects related to the pandemic. Several interesting case studies are conducting an in-depth analysis of the impact of the COVID-19 outbreak on different target groups. The management strategies and vaccine development have also been nicely explained. The interdisciplinary nature of the book makes it suitable for academicians and students belonging to science, humanities, and commerce background. The chapters are very well written and presented in an easy-to-understand manner.

Ajay Taneja
Department of Chemistry
Dr. B. R. Ambedkar University
Agra – Uttar Pradesh
India

FOREWORD II

It gives me immense pleasure to introduce the second part of the book **COVID-19: Origin, Impact and Management** ably edited by Dr. Tahmeena Khan and Dr. Alfred J. Lawrence. The book has covered many important aspects related to the COVID-19 mayhem which claimed millions of lives world over. The second part of the book has shed light on many important aspects like the effect of the pandemic on women and how they are adapting to the change in lifestyle. Not only this, but the book also includes chapters on computational drug discovery which may be useful to researchers working in medicinal chemistry. The chapters are composed and selected very ably and the authors have done a great job as all the chapters are well-written, informative and present facts in a beautiful manner.

I wish the editor great success and hope the readers would be benefitted from the enriching book.

S. H. Hasan
Department of Chemistry
IIT (BHU) Varanasi– Uttar Pradesh
India

PREFACE

The emergence of the COVID-19 pandemic was an unprecedented situation that impeded the physical and mental well-being of people globally. The expeditious discovery of vaccines and medication for decelerating the spread of SARS-CoV-2 catered to alleviating mortality rates. A comprehensive discussion on the pandemic and its impact on billions of lives has been done in part one of the two books. This part provides a meticulous overview of the COVID-19 pandemic. This book intends to collaboratively serve students, scientists and academicians from different academic areas such as science, humanities, economics; and even common masses. The collation of various heads in this book is based on contemporary needs and elaborately gives an insight into the pandemic, its impact on people's lives, especially on women, the variations that it brought in the world, and the role of air quality in exacerbating the disease. Drug discovery and vaccination hesitancy-related challenges are also scrupulously described in this book. Authors from various eminent institutions have contributed to the book which makes it a valuable collection of information. Computational Drug Discovery against the pandemic, DFT studies and molecular docking, and drug repurposing for searching potential drug candidates are the highlights of the book. Special emphasis is laid on the impact of the COVID-19 pandemic on women. The book vouches to provide a deep insight into the outbreak, epidemiology, immunology and management of SARS-CoV-2 and will be valuable for evolutionary biologists, pharmaceutical scientists and doctors. In essence, the book will supply a plethora of relevant information for degree students, research scholars, academicians, scientists and anyone who finds an interest in gathering information about the disease.

Tahmeena Khan
Department of Chemistry
Integral University
Lucknow
India

&
Alfred J. Lawrence
Department of Chemistry
Isabella Thoburn College
Lucknow
India

List of Contributors

Alfred J. Lawrence	Isabella Thoburn College, Lucknow, India
Akhilesh Kumar Maurya	University of Lucknow, Lucknow, India
Anil Mishra	University of Lucknow, Lucknow, India
Amos Nascimento	University of Washington, Tacoma/Seattle, USA
Apoorva Tandon	Krishna Institute of Engineering and Technology, Group of Institutions, Ghaziabad, India
Daraksha Bano	Integral University, Lucknow, India
Lubna Jamal	University of Lucknow, Lucknow, India
Nidhi Mishra	Indian Institute of Information Technology, Prayagraj, India
Nidhi Singh	Isabella Thoburn College, Lucknow, India
Nikita Tiwari	University of Lucknow, Lucknow, India
Rohan Srivastava	Integral University, Lucknow, India
Saima Arif	CSIR-Indian Institute of Toxicology Research (CSIR-IITR), Lucknow, India
Shristi Modanwal	Indian Institute of Information Technology, Prayagraj, India
Tahmeena Khan	Integral University, Lucknow, India
Umang Tandon	Isabella Thoburn College, Lucknow, India
Ushna Afreen	Department of Chemistry, Lucknow University, Lucknow-226007, India
Uzma Afreen	University of Lucknow, Lucknow, India
Vinay P. Aneja	North Carolina State University, USA
Viswajit Mulpuru	Indian Institute of Information Technology, Prayagraj, India

CHAPTER 1

COVID-19 Pandemic: Outbreak, Epidemiology and Immunology

Uzma Afreen[1], **Ushna Afreen**[1] and **Daraksha Bano**[2,*]

[1] *Department of Chemistry, Lucknow University, Lucknow-226007, India*

[2] *Department of Chemistry, Integral University, Lucknow-226026, India*

Abstract: The SARS-CoV-2 virus-led COVID-19 pandemic jolted the whole world at different levels. Severe acute respiratory syndrome (SARS) caused death in severe cases leading to millions of mortalities. This chapter attempts to present an overview of the whole fiasco created by the spread of the virus along with the historical background, structural features and important proteins of the virus, modes of infection and transmission and different diagnostic means like viral and antibody tests. The authors have presented the latest statistical data on the number of cases and mortalities reported across the globe and also elaborated on the probable remedial interventions like the different antiviral, antimalarial drugs which are being explored for treatment and also explored the utility and applications of drug repurposing and computational strategies for drug development. The authors have also elaborated on the different vaccines developed to curb the disease and explained the development of COVID-19 vaccines for children. Overall the chapter has summarized key facts associated with COVID-19 in a nutshell and it may prove beneficial to the readers to understand the disease more clearly.

Keywords: ACE-2, Envelope Protein, Gag-Pol Polyprotein, MERS, NAAT, Nucleocapsid Protein, OTC Tests, RT-PCR, RdRp, SARS-CoV-2, SARS, Spike Protein.

INTRODUCTION

The outbreak of the SARS-CoV-2 or COVID -19 virus has led to one of the worst pandemics in recent times. Coronaviruses (CoVs) have been recognized for over 50 years. The virologists derived the word "corona" from the sun comparing the characteristic projections on the surface of the virus with the solar corona. CoVs cause severe acute respiratory syndrome (SARS) which may lead to death in severe cases. These viruses chiefly infect human and non-human mammals and birds [1]. Coronaviruses are included in the subfamily Coronavirinae, in the

* **Corresponding author Daraksha Bano:** Department of Chemistry, Integral University, Lucknow-226026, India; E-mail: darakshab@iul.ac.in.

Tahmeena Khan & Alfred J. Lawrence (Eds.)

family Coronaviridae of the order Nidovirales [2]. Based on their phylogeny and genotype, this subfamily consists of four genera-Alphacoronavirus, Beta-coronavirus, Gammacoronavirus and Deltacoronavirus. The alphacoro-naviruses and betacoronaviruses infect only mammals, while the gammacoronaviruses and deltacoronaviruses chiefly infect birds, although some of them can also infect mammals [3]. Coronaviruses are single positive-sense RNA viruses which show greater mutation rates as compared to DNA viruses, owing to which they have better adaptation for survival. CoVs mainly affect birds and mammals. Before 2019, there were only six CoVs that were known to infect humans and caused respiratory diseases *viz*. HCoV-229E, HCoV-OC43, HCoV-NL63, HKU1, SARS-CoV and MERS-CoV. Among these, SARS-CoV and MERS-CoV have been reported to cause a severe respiratory syndrome in humans. MERS (Middle East respiratory syndrome) was first reported in Saudi Arabia in the year 2012. The COVID -19 virus, the causative agent for the coronavirus disease outbreak in 2019 emerged in Wuhan, Hubei Province, China. Wuhan, the epicentre of this virus, reported it first case in 2019. It was called Wuhan Novel Coronavirus (2019-nCoV). On the 31st of December 2019, the Chinese authorities alerted the World Health Organization (WHO) of a series of cases having pneumonia-like symptoms in the city of Wuhan. Shortly after the alert, it was recognized that the infections in humans likely originated from Huanan Seafood Market in Wuhan. After about two weeks, a team of Chinese scientists in collaboration with WHO announced that a new coronavirus (2019-nCoV), identified through genomic sequencing, was the causative agent of this pneumonia-like disease that originated in Wuhan [2]. On 9th January 2020, China declared that a novel coronavirus is the causative agent of this coronavirus disease outbreak in 2019 which is now known as COVID-19 [1]. This novel coronavirus named the severe acute respiratory syndrome coronavirus-2 (SARS-CoV-2 or 2019-nCoV) radiated from Wuhan to other areas of China. It was found to possess high homology (~80%) to the SARS-CoV [4]. The virus that causes COVID-19 (SARS-COV-2) is identified to originate in bats from where it spread to humans through contamination of meat sold in Wuhan's meat markets with wild animals' wastes [1]. By January 7th 2020, a novel beta coronavirus, SARS-CoV-2, was identified. Mortality rates are higher among people over 60 years of age and with pre-existing medical problems such as hypertension, diabetes and cardiovascular disease [5]. COVID-19 represents a spectrum of clinical manifestations encompassing fever, dry cough, fatigue and other pneumonia-like symptoms. SARS-CoV-2 is highly contagious. The mode of transmission of the disease is droplet infection and direct contact. Although respiratory droplet and contact transmission are the main transmission routes for the spread of SARS-CoV-2, aerosol and faecal-oral transmissions might also be responsible for its transmission, but have not been confirmed yet [6, 7].

HISTORICAL PERSPECTIVE

Origination of COVID-19 and Statistical Data

The ability of viruses to evolve quickly and unpredictably as they can mutate rapidly has posed great challenges to virologists. Their erratic behaviour has attracted researchers to understand their evolutionary modalities and develop strategies to subdue their activity. Many viruses have been causing various diseases in living organisms and have been, modifying their genome *via* mutation. This originates a need for continuous research on different viruses. Human viruses are distinguished based on their physical, chemical and biological properties into 26 distinct families. Coronaviridae is one of these families which includes highly infectious viruses which were earlier known to cause mild intestinal and respiratory infections in animals and humans. In the year 2002-2003, a very severe and fatal respiratory disease was encountered in Guangdong, China known as SARS which proved to be fatal. After a gap of nearly ten years another related and highly infectious strain, MERS originated in middle eastern countries where the first case was reported in the year 2012 in Jeddah, Saudi Arabia to be caused due to MERS-CoV (Middle East respiratory syndrome- coronavirus) [8]. Humans are highly susceptible to SARS-CoV and MERS-CoV (betacoronaviruses) which cause severe respiratory complications in humans. Other human coronaviruses cause mild upper respiratory tract infections with mild symptoms in adults these include HCoV-NL63, HCV-229E, HCV-OC43 and HKU1. Infants, elderly people and immunocompromised people (people with the impaired immune system) are susceptible to all the above types of human coronaviruses [3].

Later in December 2019 another fatal strain of Coronavirus came into existence in Wuhan City, China. It was named COVID-19 as it was first reported in the year 2019 [3]. A timeline of pandemics caused due to CoVs is represented in Fig. (**1**).

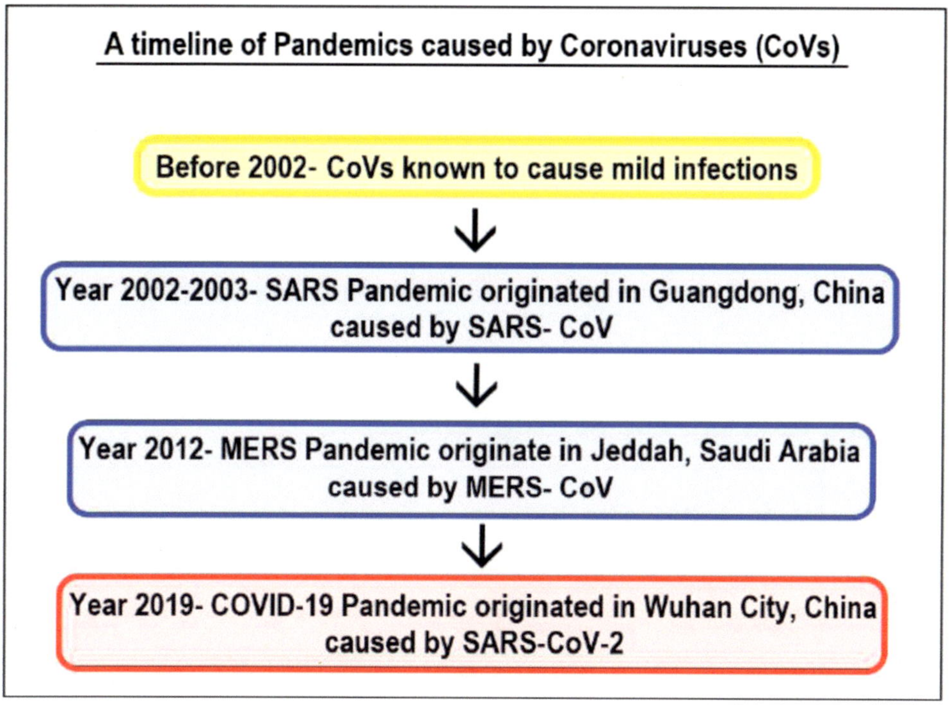

Fig. 1. Prominent Pandemics caused by CoVs.

Morphological Features of SARS-CoV-2

An insight into the morphological details of SARS-CoV-2 played an instrumental role in elucidating its mechanism of action for causing infection. The general morphology of viruses includes the genome encapsulated within a protein coat. The size of virus particles is measured in micrometres (μm) or nanometers (nm) owing to their extremely small size. The virus particle of CoV measures nearly 120 nm or 0.12 μm [9].

A coronavirus is composed of two fundamental parts:

a. The genetic material: single-stranded RNA
b. The structural proteins.

Genetic material of Coronavirus (SARS-CoV2):

The genetic material of a CoV is "enveloped positive-sense single-stranded RNA". Having RNA as the genetic material makes it possible for CoVs to mutate at a faster rate. The RNA codes for the main structural proteins of the CoVs [2, 10].

The Structural Proteins:

The structural proteins are of four types:

1. Nucleocapsid Protein (N): binds to CoV genome to make nucleocapsid.

2. Spike Protein (S): binds to ACE2 receptors on the host cell, which causes its fusion to the host cell membrane thereby making its entry into the host cell.

3. Envelope Protein (E): participates in CoV assembly and budding.

4. Membrane Protein (M): crucial for the shape of the viral envelope. It works in coordination with other major coronaviral structural proteins [11]. Fig. (**2**) represents the basic structure of SARS-CoV-2.

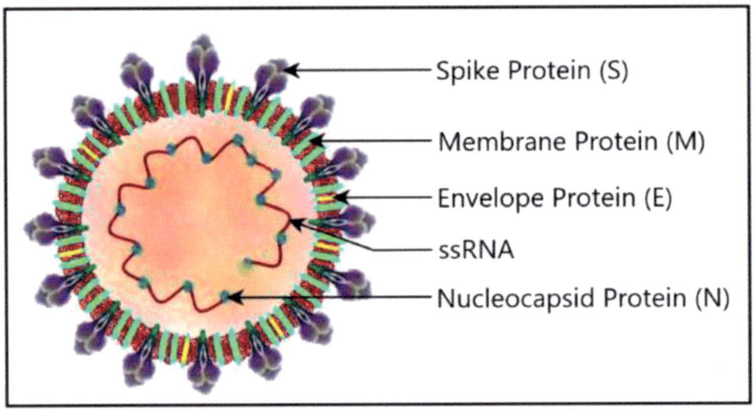

Fig. 2. Basic structure of SARS-CoV- 2.

Current Situation of COVID-19 all over the World

Soon after the onset of the COVID-19 pandemic, almost the entire globe was clutched by the SARS-CoV-2 which led to drastic life loss. Globally, as on 14th October 2022, there have been 620,878,405 confirmed cases of COVID-19, including 6,543,138 deaths, as reported by the WHO [12]. Table **1** shows the data on confirmed cases of COVID-19 in various regions worldwide.

Table 1. Data of confirmed cases of covid-19 in various regions worldwide from 3rd January 2020 to 14th October 2022*.

S.No.	Geographical Region/Area/Country	No. of Cases	No. of Deaths
1	United States of America	95,529,652	1,052,823
2	India	44,623,997	528,857
3	France	35,060,107	152,157

(Table 1) cont.....

S.No.	Geographical Region/Area/Country	No. of Cases	No. of Deaths
4	Brazil	34,736,653	687,026
5	Germany	34,517,327	151,260
6	Republic of Korea	25,076,239	28,783
7	United Kingdom	23,798,797	191,681
8	Italy	22,990,201	177,785
9	Japan	21,656,190	45,693
10	Russian Federation	21,278,816	388,709
11	Türkiye	16,919,638	101,203
12	Spain	13,441,941	114,468

*Top twelve on the basis of confirmed COVID-19 cases.

Mode of Infection

The life cycle of the virus involves the following actions: attachment, penetration, biosynthesis, maturation and release. The attachment step involves the binding of the viruses to host receptors, thereafter the SARS-CoV-2 enters the host cells by endocytosis or membrane fusion. This particular step is called penetration. Once viral contents are released inside the host cells, viral RNA invades the nucleus and the process of replication sets in. Viral mRNA translates to synthesize viral proteins. This is a crucial step and is termed biosynthesis. New viral particles are produced in the next step called maturation followed by the release of the viruses. CoVs consist of four structural proteins; Spike (S), membrane (M), envelope (E) and nucleocapsid (N) [11]. Spike is composed of a transmembrane trimetric glycoprotein projecting from the viral surface, which determines the diversity of CoVs and host tropism. Spike comprises two functional subunits; S1 and S2 which are responsible for the binding to the host cell receptor and the fusion of the viral and cellular membranes respectively. Angiotensin-converting enzyme 2 (ACE2) has been identified as the functional receptor for SARS-CoVs. Structural and functional analysis of the SARS-CoV-2 indicated that the spike protein binds to ACE2. ACE2 expression is reported to be high in the lung, heart, ileum, kidney and bladder. In the lungs, ACE2 expression of the lung epithelial cells is very high. Subsequently, the spike protein undergoes protease cleavage once the SARS-CoV-2 binds to the host protein. After the cleavage at the S1/S2 cleavage site, both the S1 and S2 subunits stay persistently bound *via* a non-covalent interaction. The distal S1 subunit contributes to the stabilization of the membrane-anchored S2 subunit at the prefusion state. Subsequent cleavage at the S2 site is presumed to activate the spike protein for membrane fusion through irreversible conformational changes. The coronavirus spike is unusual among viruses because it can be cleaved by an array of proteases [13]. The main symptoms of COVID-19 include fever, cough, fatigue, and dyspnea hence playing a key role in the early detection of this disease and early diagnosis may help in preventing the transmission of the disease to other people. About 25% of patients suffer from the presence of sputum [14]. The source of origination and transmission were important to understand to develop preventive strategies to contain the infection.

Mode of Transmission

Wild animal hosts and infected patients are currently identified as the main sources of disease which is transmitted *via* respiratory droplets and direct contact [6]. Analogous to most respiratory viruses, SARS-CoV-2 transmits predominantly *via* respiratory droplets. It is the main route, although aerosols may also be a mode of transmission. The oral-faecal route may be another route of transmission of the virus but it has not been confirmed. The stool of a patient with COVID-19 pneumonia was detected with SARS-CoV-2 RNA. This envisages that sewage might have been a source of infection of SARS-CoV-2 in humans. Moreover, the virus has also been detected in the saliva of infected individuals. This is because the epithelial cells of the salivary gland duct have receptors or target cells for the virus. The urine of some COVID-19 sufferers had also been tested for SARS-CoV-2 viral RNA [15]. A major cause for the transmission of the SARS-CoV-2 RNA is the commonly touched surfaces such as door handles, switches, and cell phones in residential sites of COVID-19-affected patients. The objects used by people in quarantine who are either positive or suspected patients are a potential cause of transmission of viable SARS-CoV-2 and lead to the spread of the virus. The analysis of the samples obtained from frequently-touched surfaces such as telephones, chairs, door handles, trolleys, *etc.* has confirmed the presence of the virus on them [16]. Bats are speculated to be the carriers of several emerging viruses including CoVs. Bats that are infected with SARS-CoV-2 have not demonstrated clinical signs of disease showing that they act as the reservoirs or ancestral hosts for several CoVs [17]. Four stages of infection have been identified: the first stage is characterised by upper respiratory tract infection; the second stage involves the onset of dyspnoea and pneumonia; the third is characterized by the worsening clinical scenario dominated by a cytokine storm and the consequent hyperinflammatory state, and the fourth stage is either death or recovery of the patient [18]. Through the sequence homology comparison at the whole-genome level in samples obtained from seven patients shared 96.2% sequence identity was observed between SARS-CoV-2 with bat-coronavirus (bat-nCoV). The intermediate host has a critical role in the transmission of SARS-CoV-2. It has been concluded through a previously reported study that the intermediate host of SARS-CoV is masked palm civet. The host receptors mediate the entry of SARS-CoV-2 *via* binding to the receptor-binding domain (RBD) of the S protein [19]. Other animals harbouring the CoVs are cattle, horses, swine, dogs, cats, camels, rabbits, rodents, birds, snakes, hedgehogs, frogs, pangolins and many other wild animals. Thus, the CoVs infect man as well as domestic and wild animal species. As is clear from the preceding discussion, among the four genera in the Coronaviridae family, Alphacoronavirus and Betacoronavirus usually infect mammals and have probable bat origin, while Gammacoronavirus and Deltacoronavirus infect birds, fishes, and mammals and are assumed to have swine origin. The SARS-CoV-2 has bats as primary hosts and palm civet cats as intermediate hosts. However, many CoVs have been recovered from birds also. The pig-infecting CoVs predominantly include Porcine Coronavirus HKU15, Transmissible Gastroenteritis Virus (TGEV), Porcine Epidemic Diarrhoea Virus (PEDV), and Porcine Hemagglutinating Encephalomyelitis virus (PHEV) [20]. From the primary host or the natural reservoir of SARS-CoV-2 *i.e.*, bats, the virus gets transmitted to the intermediate host. It then gets transmitted from the intermediate host to the human body. It is, therefore, necessary to devise measures to ensure that live-animal markets like the Huanan South China Seafood Market should be regulated by implementing strict disease-control mechanisms. Fig. (**3**) is a pictographic representation of the transmission route of the SARS-CoV-2 virus in the human population.

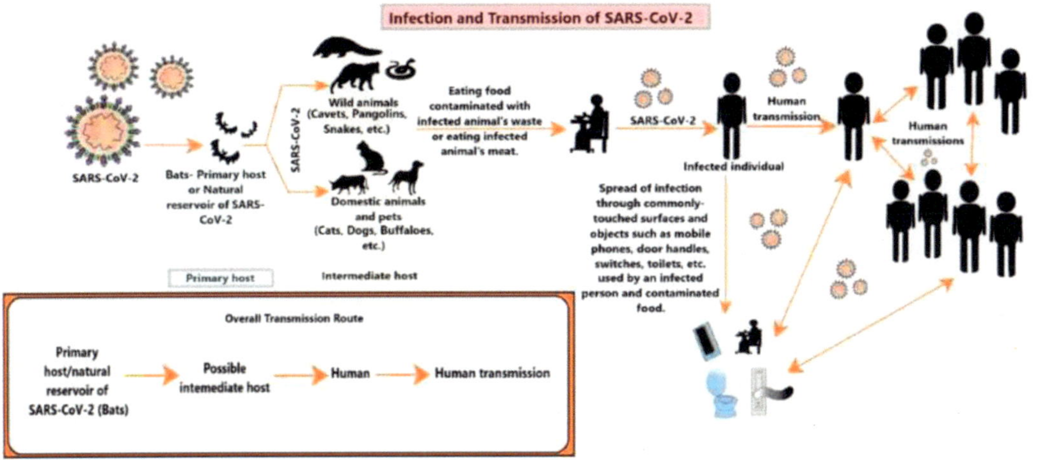

Fig. 3. A pictographic representation of the transmission of the SARS-CoV-2 virus in the human population.

Measures to Contain COVID-19

Early diagnosis of any disease is crucial for its containment. Various diagnostic techniques are employed for the detection of SARS-CoV-2. These are broadly categorised as viral and antibody tests. These diagnostic techniques along with measures taken to contain the SARS-CoV-2 are meticulously discussed in the proceeding section.

Diagnosis

The diagnosis of SARS- The coV-2 virus responsible for COVID-19 is done with the help of several clinical tests as described below:

- Viral tests

These tests find the current SARS-CoV-2 virus in samples collected for the nose or mouth of an individual. The two main types of viral tests are:

1. NAATs (Nucleic acid Amplification Tests)

One of the common NAATs is the RT-PCR (Reverse transcription-polymerase chain reaction) Test which is suitable for the detection of the genetic material of the virus. It can be employed for both symptomatic and asymptomatic individuals. Since virus genetic material stays in an individual for at least 90 days, it is advisable not to prefer this test if an individual is already tested positive in the last 90 days.

2. Antigen Test

It is a quick testing method but less reliable than RT-PCR (NAAT). It gives results in 15 minutes to 30 minutes. It can be used as a preliminary test but it is recommended to go for a NAAT for confirmation.

3. Self-Tests

These tests are antigen tests. It is done by an individual himself or herself using a self-test kit. there are various self-test kits available for purchase. It provides rapid results and is convenient option as it can be taken at any place. They test for current infection and are known as "home tests," "at-home tests," or "over-th--counter (OTC) tests". Self-tests is not useful to detect antibodies.

- **Antibody or Serology Test**

This test finds for antibody in the bloodstream that fights against the virus. This test is not preferred to diagnose current infection because it takes 1-3 weeks after the infection for the preparation of antibodies in the body [21].

PREVENTION

1. General Measures

COVID-19 spreads through respiratory droplets infection produced by infected individuals. When a healthy person comes in direct or indirect contact with infective droplets, that person also gets infected. Asymptomatic individuals can also spread the SARS-CoV-2 virus. Hence it becomes mandatory to take special preventive measures. Some of the standard operating procedures for the containment of COVID-19 are enlisted below:

- Quarantine- WHO recommended a quarantine period of 14 days if a person comes in contact with a patient suffering from COVID-19. Self-quarantine is also advisable if a person observes COVID-19 symptoms in them. Those individuals who came in contact with any symptomatic person were also adviced to avoid meeting anyone for a period of atleast 14 days so as to prevent spread of infection. Moreover, public gatherings were not allowed as a measure to prevent progression of infection in the society. People who returned from international places were made to quarantine.
- Personal hygiene- It is very important to take care of personal hygiene to prevent the spread of any disease. Hence some of the important personal hygiene measures are recommended by WHO to prevent the spread of COVID-19. One should take care of some common hygiene practices like washing hands using soap for at least twenty seconds, avoiding touching your nose, mouth and face, use sanitisers to kill viruses on your hands.
- Social distancing- As recommended by WHO physical distance of at least one meter is mandatory to avoid spreading SARS-CoV-2 [22]. As a result of this the public transport system came to a halt. People were allowed to leave their homes in their personal vehicles only in case of emergency.

2. Measures adopted by Governments all over the world

- Complete lockdown during severe pandemic conditions.
- Demarcation of certain areas as containment zones.
- Closing schools and other educational institutions completely.
- Closing offices and introducing a" work from home" strategy.
- Strict restrictions on opening marketplaces and restaurants *etc*.
- Giving guidelines for the strict use of masks when moving out of the home.
- Spraying disinfectant in public places, hospitals and residential areas.
- Expanding COVID-19 testing capacity.
- Initiating and expanding vaccination drive [23].

Probable Medicinal Intervention

Several treatments could be the first-line therapy for SARS-CoV-2 infection. These procedures have been tested on SARS-CoV-2-infected individuals. Although various vaccines having appreciable efficacy have been developed for COVID-19 but effective pharmacotherapy, including immunotherapy to avert the infection and for treatment, is yet to be established [24]. Several drugs have been used for treating COVID-19 patients. Some of these drugs and their efficacy and safety will be discussed in this section.

Antiviral Drugs

Several protease inhibitor drugs such as darunavir and atazanavir which are used for treating HIV (Human Immunodeficiency Virus) were found to inhibit the viral genome replication of SARS-CoV-2. This may be possible due to the inactivation of the proteases that are necessary to carry out replication [18, 25]. An antiviral drug, darunavir which is a nonpeptidyl HIV-1 protease inhibitor selectively inhibits Gag-Pol polyprotein cleavage resulting in immature non-infectious viral particles. Based on various *in silico* studies, darunavir has received a high score for binding with the SARS-CoV-2 protease. Thus, this drug seemed too useful for fighting the COVID-19 infection after a series of clinical testing [26] but soon a study showed that darunavir does not have antiviral effects on SARS-CoV-2 [27]. However, when it is co-administered with other antiviral drugs, it showed good results in treating SARS-CoV-2 patients [25, 28]. A study reported that immunocompromised patients having HIV infections do not get protection from SARS-CoV-2 infection by the use of darunavir [29]. Yet, darunavir showed potential effectiveness when co-administered with other antivirals. Oseltamivir is another antiviral drug which is known to inhibit neuraminidase. It is used to block influenza A and B viruses. The neuraminidase enzyme is essential for the entry of the virus to the host cell, the release of the virus from the host cells and the further spread of infection in the entire body. Being a neuraminidase inhibitor, oseltamivir prevents the release of viruses by keeping them attached to the membrane of the previously infected host cells thereby preventing the expansion of the infection. In combination with Lopinavir and Ritonavir, Oseltamivir reduced symptoms in SARS-CoV-2-infected individuals. The synergistic effects of lopinavir, ritonavir and oseltamivir have been studied *in silico*, and it was found that the co-administration of these three drugs has high effectiveness against SARS-CoV-2 protease. Oseltamivir alone cannot prevent COVID-19 as SARS-CoV-2 lacks neuraminidase [25]. A broad-spectrum antiviral, Umifenovir is an anti-influenza drug that was also approved for its use against SARS-CoV in 2004. Due to its broad-spectrum antiviral activities, Umifenovir had been proposed as an efficient drug for treating COVID-19 but its monotherapy did not improve patients' conditions and no alleviation in the symptoms of COVID-19 was observed [25]. Favipiravir which is an anti-RNA antiviral drug incorporates viral RNA through substitution with purines. This leads to the inhibition of RNA-dependent RNA polymerase of the virus thereby preventing RNA elongation. The RNA structure of SARS-CoV-2 and its similarities to SARS-CoV make Favipiravir a potential drug candidate for treating COVID-19 patients [25, 30]. Various reviews reveal that favipiravir shows faster viral clearance compared to co-administered Lopinavir/Ritonavir and Umifenovir [31]. Another potential drug molecule, remdesivir, had shown commendable activity against SARS-CoV-2. it is a small molecule monophosphoramidate prodrug. Remdesivir is an adenosine analogue and blocks the RNA-dependent RNA polymerase (RdRp). Remdesivir is cleaved to the nucleoside monophosphate analogue and undergoes phosphorylation yielding an active remdesivir triphosphate (RDV-TP) form resembling the adenosine triphosphate (ATP). Thus, it competes with ATP and gets incorporated into the viral RNA. This helps in the premature termination of the viral RNA transcription resulting in the inhibition of RNA synthesis [25, 32]. *In vitro* and *in vivo* experiments on SARS-CoV and MERS-CoV showed that Remdesivir could inhibit the viruses' replication and reduces viral lung load and SARS-CoV-induced lung pathology such as denuding bronchiolitis. The studies on the half-maximal effective concentration (EC50) and half-cytotoxic effective concentration (CC50) of remdesivir revealed that it can show sufficient inhibition activity for SARS-CoV-2 [33]. On the 1st of May, 2020, FDA (U.S. Food and Drug Administration) authorized remdesivir for emergency use for treating hospitalized COVID-19 patients. However, for the covid-19 patients having mild or moderate symptoms, remdesivir is not recommended. For those patients who require respiratory support, the use of remdesivir is recommended for a speedy recovery and to alleviate the hazard of the spread of SARS-CoV-2 in the other body cells [25, 34]. Ribavirin is another anti-viral that leads to viral RNA degradation. However, the majority of reports on SARS CoV and MERS CoV suggest that Ribavirin can be an add-on therapy as a combination with Lopinavir/Ritonavir or interferon [35].

Antibacterial Drugs

Various antibacterial drugs such as teicoplanin and azithromycin have also been tested for their efficacy against COVID-19. Teicoplanin, a glycopeptide antibiotic, is reported to be potentially appropriate for the treatment of COVID-19 [36]. Azithromycin has been reported to show no positive effects against SARS-CoV-2 [25]. The antibacterial drugs have not shown positive results against SARS-CoV-2 as their efficacy was found to be too low.

Antimalarial Drugs

Antimalarial agents- chloroquine and hydroxychloroquine were also assessed for their activity against SARS-CoV-2 but were found to be non-beneficial as announced by FDA in June 2020 [25].

Immunomodulatory Drugs

Several immunomodulatory drugs also went through numerous experiments and clinical tests. The most used immunomodulatory drug in the treatment of COVID-19 was Tocilizumab. Baricitinib is another immunomodulator that had been suggested as a possible therapy for COVID-19. Although it was used only during the early phase of COVID-19 disease [18].

Monoclonal Antibodies

As reported in previous studies, monoclonal antibodies against specific cytokines and corticosteroids appear to be useful in improving clinical conditions in patients with critical-stage COVID-19 [18].

Thus, it may be inferred that the antiviral agents are most useful to suppress the clinical progression and problems associated with COVID-19. However, there is still a need to identify specific targets that inhibit the life cycle of SARS-CoV-2 to prevent viral genome replication. Studies have shown clinical and survival improvement in COVID-19 patients who were treated with plasma and hyperimmune immunoglobulins. Inflammation inhibitors are quite valuable for the treatment of COVID-19 in its advanced stages. A series of clinical trials are required to further confirm the safety and efficacy of these drug candidates, and determine which stage of COVID-19 is most appropriate to administer the drugs to achieve the best results concerning disease regression.

Drug Repurposing and Computational Assessment

Many drugs that were earlier used for treating other diseases have been used as a medical intervention for COVID-19 patients and proved to be very helpful in controlling emergencies. Remdesivir is considered the most potent drug against the SARS-CoV-2 [37]. Remdesivir, a nucleotide analogue prodrug, perturbs viral replication and was originally evaluated in clinical trials to prevent the Ebola outbreak in 2014. Assessment of the drug through numerous virology laboratory tests demonstrated its ability to inhibit SARS-CoV-2 genome replication [38]. This drug-repurposing has been possible due to computational assessment of pre-existing drugs used for treating other diseases. Drug repurposing appreciably reduced the time, cost, and risks of finding possible medication for COVID-19 as compared to developing new drug candidates. The assessment of the effectiveness of available FDA-approved drugs made it possible to rapidly develop eligible drugs to treat COVID-19. The *in silico* studies helped to construct a covalent bond with Cys145 inside the binding site SARS-CoV-2 main protease by using covalent docking screening. The covalent docking revealed that various drugs such as saquinavir, ritonavir, remdesivir, delavirdine, oseltamivir and a few others show high binding energies. Therefore, *in silico* techniques have been powerful tools for determining drug interactions with the binding site and acted as a means for rapid screening of drugs. This led to the quick availability of drugs that can be used in the treatment of SARS-CoV-2 [39].

Vaccines and Futuristic Strategies

Ensuring the emergence of novel betacoronavirus SARS-CoV-2, in December 2019, a quest for developing a successful vaccine was initiated. as a result of this explosion of vaccine development, by the September 24th, 2020, an astonishing number of vaccines went into pre-trial development. These were 200 vaccines out of which 43 entered clinical trials [40]. On account of the unfettered cases and deaths of people, it was imperative to develop a vaccine as early as possible. The fastest any vaccine had been developed previously successfully was in 4 years and this vaccine was for mumps in the 1960s. It was quite a daunting task for the researchers to develop a vaccine faster than this. Yet the beginning of December 2021 marked the successful development of the first vaccine for emergency use for SARS-CoV-2, the first fully tested immunization to be approved for emergency use was a vaccine made by Pfizer with German biotech firm BioNTech. New ways were employed for vaccine development such as the use of messenger RNA (mRNA). This fast development of a vaccine in 18 months ignited hopes that the vaccine development process for other diseases can also be accelerated manifold by working on the same lines. It has been possible to develop COVID-19 vaccines so quickly because of years of previous research on related viruses as well as advanced fast methods for manufacturing vaccines and enormous funding. For years, researchers had been studying coronaviruses, which cause SARS and MERS. It takes years to develop fully functional and safe vaccines, but scientists created multiple vaccines for SARS-CoV-2 in the short duration of a year. Conventional vaccines contain viral proteins or disabled forms of the virus itself, which stimulate the body's immune system against infection by a live virus. But the case of the first two COVID-19 vaccines that were announced in large-scale (phase III) clinical trials involved merely an mRNA strand enclosed in a lipid layer. The mRNA encodes a protein of SARS-CoV-2. When this mRNA enters the body cells, the corresponding protein synthesis gets initiated. This protein acts as the antigen (the cause of virulence) that triggers the body's immune response. The vaccines that were developed by Pfizer and BioNTech and by the US pharmaceutical company Moderna utilized mRNA that codes for the spike protein of the SARS-CoV-2, which anchors to human cell membranes and allows the coronavirus to invade the cell [41].

Vaccines are typically divided into several types *viz*., inactivated vaccines, live attenuated vaccines, vectored vaccines, nucleic acid-based vaccines, and recombinant subunit vaccines. Inactivated and live attenuated vaccines are based on the antigenicity of a killed and weakened virus, respectively. Vectored vaccines use other viruses as vectors for SARS-CoV-2 proteins. In case of the nucleic acid-based vaccines, the injection of nucleic acid is given to the patient which expresses the viral genes and can result in the activation of both humoral and cellular immune responses. Recombinant subunit vaccines are composed of several microbial components produced in a heterologous expression system [42]. Various successful COVID-19 vaccines have been developed using either of these approaches and have been discussed herein.

RNA-Based Vaccines

BNT162b2 is an RNA-based vaccine which has approximately 82% efficacy with the first dose which increases to nearly 95% after the second dose in the symptomatic COVID-19 patients. mRNA-1273 is another RNA-based vaccine for COVID-19 which shows around 94% efficacy after two doses. CVnCoV is yet another RNA-based vaccine but its efficacy is low (approximately 48%). ChAdOx1 nCoV-19 vaccine shows an average efficacy of 70%.

Viral Vector Vaccines

Some non-replicating viral vector vaccines such as AZD1222, Ad26.COV2.S, ConvideciAd5-nCoV and Gam-COVID-Vax Sputnik V have also been employed for vaccinating people against COVID-19. The Gam-COVID-Vax Sputnik V has 63.7-80.1% efficacy with the first dose and 85.6- 95.2% efficacy with the second dose.

Protein-Based Vaccines

NVX-CoV2373 and Abdala are protein-based vaccines used to vaccinate people against COVID-19. Out of these two, Abdala shows 92.3% efficacy which is quite higher than that of NVX-CoV2373 (approximately 89%).

Inactivated Virus Vaccines

CoronaVac, BBIBP-CorV and COVAXIN are prepared from inactivated SARS-CoV-2. CoronaVac shows low efficacy of approximately 50%. COVAXIN is prepared by Bharat biotech and shows approximately 78% efficacy [43].

In a nutshell, it can be said that the fastest vaccine development to date has been the development of a vaccine for SARS-CoV-2. This successful fast development can be of the vaccine is attributed to the years of research on related viruses. Various vaccines developed to date against COVID-19 used various approaches and showed significant efficacy. Table **2** shows the number of vaccinations done in some regions of the world [12]. However, there was a need to develop vaccines that are safe for children too.

Table 2. -Number of vaccine doses administered for covid-19.

S.No.	Geographical Region/Area/Country	Till Date	No. of Doses
1	United States of America	6th OCTOBER 2022	616,508,199
2	India	11th OCTOBER 2022	2,190,969,572
3	France	1st OCTOBER 2022	152,968,321
4	Brazil	6th OCTOBER 2022	484,474,086
5	Germany	1st OCTOBER 2022	185,704,376
6	Republic of Korea	29th SEPTEMBER 2022	130,834,289
7	United Kingdom	3rd SEPTEMBER 2022	151,248,820
8	Italy	1st OCTOBER 2022	139,669,852
9	Japan	15th SEPTEMBER 2022	321,037,169
10	Russian Federation	11th OCTOBER 2022	178,107,276
11	Türkiye	10th OCTOBER 2022	152,318,861
12	Spain	1st OCTOBER 2022	103,045,916

COVID-19 Vaccines for Children

The development of the pediatric COVID-19 vaccine was another big challenge. In May 2021, Canada became the first country to approve the COVID-19 vaccine for emergency use in children of age 12 to 15. Later, in May 2021, the US Food and Drug Administration and European medicines Agency also approved the Pfizer-BioNTech COVID-19 vaccine for the age group 12-15. For children of age 3 to 17, the inactivated vaccine CoronaVac was found safe and showed good immunogenicity. other COVID-19 vaccines are under trails for their safety in children. The BNT162b2 COVID-19 vaccine was evaluated for its use in children between 5-11 years of age. The safe dosage had to be determined and its efficacy against COVID-19 had to be evaluated. In a study conducted in the year 2022, it was found that no vaccine-related critical adverse effects were noted in 5 to 11 years old children. It consisted of two 10μg doses of BNT162b2 administered in a gap of 21 days and were found safe, immunogenic, and efficacious in the age group [44]. In the year 2021, on October 29th, FDA amended the Emergency Use

Authorization (EUA) for Pfizer-BioNTech COVID-19 (BNT162b2) mRNA vaccine to expand its use to 5 to 11 years old children. Its administration is done in two doses (10 µg, 0.2mL each) in a gap of 21 days (3 weeks). By December 19, 2021, it was only the Pfizer-BioNTech COVID-19 vaccine which was authorized to be safe for administration to children aged 5–17 years [45]. No severe and life-threatening effects are reported due to COVID-19 vaccination in children. Fig. (**4**) shows a comparison between some COVID-19 vaccines.

A comparison of some COVID-19 vaccines

Vaccine	Type	Doses	Efficacy
BNT162b2 (Pfizer & BioNTech)	RNA	2	95%
mRNA-1273 (Moderna)	RNA	2	94%
Gam-COVID-Vax Sputnik V	Viral vector	2	92%
NVX-CoV2373 (Novavax	Protein-based	2	89%
ChAdox1 nCoV (University of Oxford or AstraZeneca	Viral vector	2	70%
CoronaVac (Sinovac)	Inactivated virus	2	50%

Fig. 4. A comparison between some COVID-19 vaccines.

CONCLUSION

There's no doubt that the flare-up of COVID-19 shook the entire world. As of 19th October 2022, 6,573,890 people have died due to COVID-19. The data obtained till 19th October reported 630,707,049 confirmed cases in 228 countries and territories across the globe. However, 609,836,590 patients recovered from the disease as of 19th October 2022. There are 14,296,569 currently infected patients out of which 14,257,832 (99.7%) are in mild condition while 38,737 (0.3%) are having serious or critical conditions, as of 19th October 2022. There were 616,410,480 cases which had an outcome- 609,836,590 (99%) recovered while 6,573,890 (1%) died. Bearing in mind that a large number of cases have been either asymptomatic or present with very mild symptoms and that testing has not been performed on the entire population, only a fraction of the SARS-CoV-2 infected population is detected confirmed through a laboratory test, and officially reported as a COVID-19 case. Therefore, the exact number of COVID-19 cases by far is not known. However, it might be considered to be at several multiples above the presently reported number of cases. The number of deaths that have occurred globally also tends to be underestimated, as some patients were not hospitalized and did not even get tested [46]. Globally there have been about 3.4% of reported COVID-19 cases have died. As compared to the seasonal flu which generally kills far fewer than 1% of infected individuals [47]. The officially accepted incubation period of SARS-CoV-2 is 2 - 14 days. The death rates were greater for older people (60 years and above age) as compared to young people. The death rate for male patients was also found higher than that for females [48]. Patients suffering from COVID-19 have a wide range of symptoms including-fever, cough, shortness of breath or difficulty in breathing, chills, muscle pain, headache, sore throat, and loss of taste or smell [49]. The most common symptoms that were reported in most of the patients were fever, cough, fatigue, and dyspnea [14]. The recovery of 609,836,590 patients indicates that the vaccination drive, social distancing, drugs used to treat COVID-19 and other preventive measures have been quite successful. However, as discussed in the preceding sections, researchers are still in search of powerful prevention and remediation strategies for the SARS-CoV-2 virus. The development of vaccines such as Pfizer and BioNTech, Moderna, Sputnik V and others had led to a dramatic decrease in the number of new cases of COVID-19. Drugs like remdesivir have played a vital role in alleviating symptoms of patients and saved the lives of many people who were suffering from COVID-19 infection. Vaccination along with social awareness played a key role in diminishing the progression rate of the SARS-COV-2 virus. The proper implementation of the Government guidelines would further alleviate the number of cases to zero as they have already pulled down the number from lakhs to a few thousand. The development of vaccines for COVID-19 has by far been the fastest only after the Mumps vaccine. It was a wonderful achievement for researchers throughout the world who worked on COVID-19 vaccine development as it helped in preventing the spread of infection to a great extent.

CONSENT FOR PUBLICATION

Not applicable.

CONFLICT OF INTEREST

The authors declare no conflict of interest, financial or otherwise.

ACKNOWLEDGEMENTS

Declared none.

REFERENCES

[1] Hamed MA. An overview on COVID-19: reality and expectation. Bull Natl Res Cent 2020; 44(1): 86. [http://dx.doi.org/10.1186/s42269-020-00341-9] [PMID: 32514228]

[2] Seah I, Su X, Lingam G. Revisiting the dangers of the coronavirus in the ophthalmology practice. Eye (Lond) 2020; 34(7): 1155-7. [http://dx.doi.org/10.1038/s41433-020-0790-7] [PMID: 32029919]

[3] Cui J, Li F, Shi ZL. Origin and evolution of pathogenic coronaviruses. Nat Rev Microbiol 2019; 17(3): 181-92. [http://dx.doi.org/10.1038/s41579-018-0118-9] [PMID: 30531947]

[4] Yuki K, Fujiogi M, Koutsogiannaki S. COVID-19 pathophysiology: A review. Clin Immunol 2020; 215: 108427. [http://dx.doi.org/10.1016/j.clim.2020.108427] [PMID: 32325252]

[5] Cevik M, Bamford C G G, Ho A. COVID-19 pandemic- a focussed review for clinicians. Narrative Review 2020; 26(7): 842. [http://dx.doi.org/10.1016/j.cmi.2020.04.023]

[6] Shi Y, Wang G, Cai X, *et al.* An overview of COVID-19. J Zhejiang University-SCIENCE B (Biomedicine & Biotechnology) 2020; 21(5): 343-7. [http://dx.doi.org/10.1631/jzus.B2000083]

[7] Ndwandwe D, Wiysonge CS. COVID-19 vaccines. Curr Opin Immunol 2021; 71: 111-6. [http://dx.doi.org/10.1016/j.coi.2021.07.003] [PMID: 34330017]

[8] 2020.https://apps.who.int/iris/bitstream/handle/10665/332197/WHO-2019-nCoV-FAQ-Virus_orgin-2020.1-eng.pdf

[9] 2022.https://www.britannica.com/science/coronavirus-virus-group

[10] V'kovski P, Kratzel A, Steiner S, Stalder H, Thiel V. Coronavirus biology and replication: implications for SARS-CoV-2. Nat Rev Microbiol 2021; 19(3): 155-70. [http://dx.doi.org/10.1038/s41579-020-00468-6] [PMID: 33116300]

[11] Schoeman D, Fielding BC. Coronavirus envelope protein: current knowledge. Virol J 2019; 16(1): 69. [http://dx.doi.org/10.1186/s12985-019-1182-0] [PMID: 31133031]

[12] 2022.https://covid19.who.int/

[13] Yuki K, Fujiogi M, Koutsogiannaki S. COVID-19 pathophysiology: A review. Clin Immunol 2020; 215: 108427. [http://dx.doi.org/10.1016/j.clim.2020.108427] [PMID: 32325252]

[14] Alimohamadi Y, Sepandi M, Taghdir M, Hosamirudsari H. Determine the most common clinical symptoms in COVID-19 patients: a systematic review and meta-analysis. J Prev Med Hyg 2020; 61(3): E304-12. [http://dx.doi.org/10.15167%2F2421-4248%2Fjpmh2020.61.3.1530] [PMID: 33150219]

[15] Ciotti M, Ciccozzi M, Terrinoni A, *et al.* The COVID-19 pandemic Critical Reviews in Clinical Laboratory Sciences 2020; 57(6): 367. [http://dx.doi.org/10.1080/10408363.2020.1783198]

[16] Dargahi A, Jeddi F, Vosoughi M, *et al.* Investigation of SARS CoV-2 virus in environmental surface. Environ Res 2021; 195: 110765. [http://dx.doi.org/10.1016/j.envres.2021.110765] [PMID: 33497684]

[17] Banerjee A, Kulcsar K, Misra V, Frieman M, Mossman K. Bats and Coronaviruses. Viruses 2019; 11(1): 41. [http://dx.doi.org/10.3390/v11010041] [PMID: 30634396]

[18] Stasi C, Fallani S, Voller F, Silvestri C. Treatment for COVID-19: An overview. Eur J Pharmacol

2020; 889: 173644.
[http://dx.doi.org/10.1016/j.ejphar.2020.173644] [PMID: 33053381]

[19] Zhao J, Cui W, Tian B. The Potential Intermediate Hosts for SARS-CoV-2. Front Microbiol 2020; 11: 580137.
[http://dx.doi.org/10.3389/fmicb.2020.580137] [PMID: 33101254]

[20] Tiwari R, Dhama K, Sharun K, *et al.* COVID-19: animals, veterinary and zoonotic links. Vet Q 2020; 40(1): 169-82.
[http://dx.doi.org/10.1080/01652176.2020.1766725] [PMID: 32393111]

[21] 2022.https://www.cdc.gov/coronavirus/2019-ncov/symptoms-testing/testing.html

[22] 2022.https://www.who.int/emergencies/diseases/novel-coronavirus-2019/advice-for-public

[23] Güner R, Hasanoğlu İ, Aktaş F. COVID-19: Prevention and control measures in community. Turk J Med Sci 2020; 50(SI-1): 571-7.
[http://dx.doi.org/10.3906/sag-2004-146] [PMID: 32293835]

[24] Paudyal V, Sun S, Hussain R, Abutaleb MH, Hedima EW. Complementary and alternative medicines use in COVID-19: A global perspective on practice, policy and research. Res Social Adm Pharm 2022; 18(3): 2524-8.
[http://dx.doi.org/10.1016/j.sapharm.2021.05.004] [PMID: 33992585]

[25] Tarighi P, Eftekhari S, Chizari M, Sabernavaei M, Jafari D, Mirzabeigi P. A review of potential suggested drugs for coronavirus disease (COVID-19) treatment. Eur J Pharmacol 2021; 895: 173890.
[http://dx.doi.org/10.1016/j.ejphar.2021.173890] [PMID: 33482181]

[26] Pant S, Singh M, Ravichandiran V, Murty USN, Srivastava HK. Peptide-like and small-molecule inhibitors against Covid-19. J Biomol Struct Dyn 2021; 39(8): 2904-13.
[http://dx.doi.org/10.1080/07391102.2020.1757510] [PMID: 32306822]

[27] De Meyer S, Bojkova D, Cinatl J, *et al.* Lack of antiviral activity of darunavir against SARS-CoV-2. Int J Infect Dis 2020; 97: 7-10.
[http://dx.doi.org/10.1016/j.ijid.2020.05.085] [PMID: 32479865]

[28] Costanzo M, De Giglio MAR, Roviello GN. SARS CoV-2: recent reports on antiviral therapies based on lopinavir/ritonavir, darunavir/umifenovir, hydroxychloroquine, remdesivir, favipiravir and other drugs for the treatment of the new coronavirus (2020). Curr Med Chem 2020; 27(27): 4536-41.
[http://dx.doi.org/10.2174/1875533XMTA1tODYl1] [PMID: 32297571]

[29] Riva A, Conti F, Bernacchia D, *et al.* Darunavir does not prevent SARS-CoV-2 infection in HIV patients. Pharmacol Res 2020; 157: 104826.
[http://dx.doi.org/10.1016/j.phrs.2020.104826] [PMID: 32325127]

[30] Du YX, Chen XP. Favipiravir: pharmacokinetics and concerns about clinical trials for 2019-nCoV infection. Clin Pharmacol Ther 2020; 108(2): 242-7.
[http://dx.doi.org/10.1002/cpt.1844] [PMID: 32246834]

[31] Siordia JA Jr, Bernaba M, Yoshino K, *et al.* Systematic and statistical review of coronavirus disease 19 treatment trials. SN Compr Clin Med 2020; 2(8): 1120-31.
[http://dx.doi.org/10.1007/s42399-020-00399-6] [PMID: 32838169]

[32] Khanal P. Remdesivir for COVID-19 treatment: mechanism OF action, synthesis, and clinical trials. J Pharm Pharm Sci 2020; 9: 8.
[http://dx.doi.org/10.20959/wjpps20208-16808]

[33] Wang M, Cao R, Zhang L, *et al.* Remdesivir and chloroquine effectively inhibit the recently emerged novel coronavirus (2019-nCoV) *in vitro*. Cell Res 2020; 30(3): 269-71.
[http://dx.doi.org/10.1038/s41422-020-0282-0] [PMID: 32020029]

[34] Young B, Tan TT, Leo YS. The place for remdesivir in COVID-19 treatment. Lancet Infect Dis 2021; 21(1): 20-1.

[http://dx.doi.org/10.1016/S1473-3099(20)30911-7] [PMID: 33248473]

[35] Song Y, Zhang M, Yin L, *et al.* COVID-19 treatment: close to a cure? A rapid review of pharmacotherapies for the novel coronavirus (SARS-CoV-2). Int J Antimicrob Agents 2020; 56(2): 106080.
[http://dx.doi.org/10.1016/j.ijantimicag.2020.106080]

[36] Ceccarelli G, Alessandri F, d'Ettorre G, *et al.* Is teicoplanin a complementary treatment option for COVID-19? The question remains. Int J Antimicrob Agents 2020; 56(2): 106029.
[http://dx.doi.org/10.1016/j.ijantimicag.2020.106029] [PMID: 32454071]

[37] Jean SS, Hsueh PR. Old and re-purposed drugs for the treatment of COVID-19. Expert Rev Anti Infect Ther 2020; 18(9): 843-7.
[http://dx.doi.org/10.1080/14787210.2020.1771181] [PMID: 32419524]

[38] Eastman RT, Roth JS, Brimacombe KR, *et al.* Remdesivir: A Review of Its Discovery and Development Leading to Emergency Use Authorization for Treatment of COVID-19. ACS Cent Sci 2020; 6(5): 672-83.
[http://dx.doi.org/10.1021/acscentsci.0c00489] [PMID: 32483554]

[39] Al-Khafaji K, AL-Duhaidahawi D, Taskin Tok T. Using integrated computational approaches to identify safe and rapid treatment for SARS-CoV-2. J Biomol Struct Dyn 2020; 39(9): 1-9.
[http://dx.doi.org/10.1080/07391102.2020.1764392] [PMID: 32364041]

[40] Tregoning JS, Brown ES, Cheeseman HM, *et al.* Vaccines for COVID-19. Clin Exp Immunol 2020; 202(2): 162-92.
[http://dx.doi.org/10.1111/cei.13517] [PMID: 32935331]

[41] Ball P. The lightning-fast quest for COVID vaccines — and what it means for other diseases. Nature 2021; 589(7840): 16-8.
[http://dx.doi.org/10.1038/d41586-020-03626-1] [PMID: 33340018]

[42] Dhi Yu, Wang G, Cai X, *et al.* An overview of COVID-19 (2020). J Zhejiang University-SCIENCE B (Biomedicine & Biotechnology); 21(5):353-354.
[http://dx.doi.org/10.1631/jzus.B2000083]

[43] Fiolet T, Kherabi Y, MacDonald CJ, Ghosn J, Peiffer-Smadja N. Comparing COVID-19 vaccines for their characteristics, efficacy and effectiveness against SARS-CoV-2 and variants of concern: a narrative review. Clin Microbiol Infect 2022; 28(2): 202-21.
[http://dx.doi.org/10.1016/j.cmi.2021.10.005] [PMID: 34715347]

[44] Walter EB, Talaat KR, Sabharwal C, *et al.* Evaluation of the BNT162b2 Covid-19 Vaccine in Children 5 to 11 Years of Age. N Engl J Med 2022; 386(1): 35-46.
[http://dx.doi.org/10.1056/NEJMoa2116298] [PMID: 34752019]

[45] Hause AM, Baggs J, Marquez P, *et al.* COVID-19 Vaccine Safety in Children Aged 5–11 Years — United States, November 3–December 19, 2021. MMWR Morb Mortal Wkly Rep 2021; 70(5152): 1755-60.
[http://dx.doi.org/10.15585/mmwr.mm705152a1] [PMID: 34968370]

[46] 2022.https://www.worldometers.info/coronavirus/coronavirus death-rate/#ref-13

[47] 2020.https://www.who.int/director-general/speeches/detail/who-director-general-s-opening-r-marks-at-the-media-briefing-on-covid-19---3-march-2020

[48] 2022.https://www.worldometers.info/coronavirus/coronavirus-age-sex-demographics/

[49] 2022.https://www.worldometers.info/coronavirus/coronavirus-symptoms/

CHAPTER 2

The Impact of Air Pollution and Environmental Factors on COVID-19 Transmission

Alfred J. Lawrence[1], **Vinay P. Aneja**[2] and **Tahmeena Khan**[3,*]

[1] *Department of Chemistry, Isabella Thoburn College, Lucknow, India*

[2] *North Carolina State University, USA*

[3] *Department of Chemistry, Integral University, Lucknow, India*

Abstract: SARS-CoV-2 (COVID-19) has caused serious mortal damage to the human race. The virus causes respiratory infections, and many studies are trying to comprehend the mode of spread and infection. This chapter has explained the origin of the virus, its structure and activity domain, symptoms, medicinal interventions, and particularly various modes of spread with emphasis on air pollution as contributing and facilitating factors assisted with favourable meteorological conditions, including temperature and relative humidity. Pieces of evidence from different countries suggest that the spread of the virus may be facilitated by air pollution and people who are exposed to high pollution levels are more susceptible to falling victim to the virus. Transmission of the SARS-CoV-2 may be facilitated by the airborne particulate matter, and both particulate matter and coronavirus cause oxidative stress in the body that helps in enhancing the susceptibility and severity towards respiratory infection. Not only ambient air pollution, but indoor air pollution (IAP) is also a factor worth considering. People in developing and under-developed nations are at high risk as they are exposed to high IAP levels. Awareness must be created to educate them about the associated harmful consequences, including the risk of catching the lethal COVID-19 infection. In the absence of any concrete medicinal solution, it is necessary to build immunity which may be uplifted by the usage of natural food sources, including herbs and spices. An overview of some commonly available herbs and spices of medicinal importance has also been given in the chapter.

Keywords: Air Pollution, Airborne , Environment, Humidity, Indoor Pollution, Oxidative Stress, Particulate matter, Respiratory Infection, SARS-CoV-2, Temperature.

* **Corresponding author Tahmeena Khan**: Department of Chemistry, Integral University, Lucknow, India; E-mail: tahminakhan30@yahoo.com

INTRODUCTION

The outbreak of Severe Acute Respiratory Syndrome coronavirus (SARS-CoV-2) has surfaced as a major health concern all over the world [1]. The outbreak was pronounced a health emergency on 30th January 2020, and subsequently, on 11 March 2020, the WHO declared COVID-19 a pandemic. The coronavirus was first isolated in the year 1965 by Tyrrell and Bynoe from a child with a cold and flu and termed B814 [2]. The term coronavirus was coined owing to the morphological characteristics of the virus in the year 1968 [3]. The virus may be transmitted through, 1) direct contact with the infected person, 2) aerosol generation and inhalation by a healthy person and 3) environmental factors [4]. It has been found that dried SARS-CoV-2 can be viable for 3-4 days at room temperature between 22-25 ^{0}C for 14 days at a temperature of 4 ^{0}C but becomes inactive at a warm temperature. The live virus has been cultured from aerosols and surfaces even after hours of inoculation, but strong evidence suggests respiratory transmission with closeness to the infected patient and ventilation being the key determinants [5]. The viral spike protein (S) binds to the angiotensin-converting enzyme 2 (ACE2) receptor, which is crucial for the entry of the pathogen into the host cell and the distribution of ACE2 [6]. The viral load is highest in the upper respiratory tract initially and later on reaches the lower respiratory tract (sputum). It has also been found that susceptibility to infection increases with age [7]. A study from Iceland reported 6.7% and 13.7% positivity in children and adults, and 4% and 17.1% positivity was obtained from Wuhan, China [8]. Low expression of ACE2 in children may be responsible for the difference in positivity rate [9].

HISTORICAL PERSPECTIVE

The novel coronavirus that causes COVID-19 has been linked to animals and was reportedly transmitted to humans in Wuhan, China, in December 2019 [10]. To date, all coronaviruses causing human infection originated from bats or rodents [11]. In the year 2007, scientists from Hong Kong brought to notice the emergence and re-emergence of SARS [11]. The US Centers for Disease Control and Prevention (2017) estimates that three-quarters of new or emerging diseases that infect humans originate in animals [12]. Outbreaks of previously known SARS-CoV and MERS-CoV involved exposure to other animals like civet cats and dromedary camels. The virus appears as a crown with petal-like projections protruding from the surface, thereby acquiring the Latin name “corona” meaning crown [13]. They are positive-sense RNA viruses belonging to the Coronavirinae subfamily of the order Nidovirales [14] and are categorized as alpha, beta, gamma and delta based on their genomic structure. Out of which, the first two cause respiratory symptoms in mammals [15].

Two major outbreaks caused by coronaviruses, 1- SARS in 2003 caused 1,000, and 2- Middle East Respiratory Syndrome (MERS) in 2012 led to 862 fatalities. The SARS incidence was first reported in late 2002 and reemerged in late 2003 [16] due to an interspecies transmission. The viral outbreak was first reported in China, where the increasing demand for animal proteins, including civets, led to their bearing in close confinements, and in the absence of biosafety measures, the virus spread like an epidemic from animals to humans, later from person to person transmission [17]. The virus is zoonotic because of its transmission from animals to humans [18]. The SARS coronaviruses are characterized by spike proteins containing a variable receptor-binding domain (RBD) which binds to the ACE-2 receptor [19], facilitating viral entry in the target cells. The RBD of SARS-CoV-2 seems to be a mutant of RaTG13, a virus sampled from bats [20], thereby showing that the virus originated from bats. Until December 2019, six coronaviruses were identified to cause infection in humans. HCoV-NL63, HCoV-229E, HCoV-OC43 and HKU1 were responsible for causing mild cold-type symptoms in people with compromised immunity, and the other two led to pandemics during the last two decades.

Facts and Figures

WHO has characterized the transmission as 1- Nations with no reported cases, 2- Infrequent cases, 3-Clusters of cases, 4- Community transmission [20]. From 31st December 2019 to 21st January 2022, 340543962 cases have been reported with 5570163 casualties (European Centre for Disease Prevention and Control (ECDC) 2022). With time, the virus changes its properties like the spread, severity of infection, therapeutic interventions, diagnostic methods and other public health measures. WHO has been in the process of assessing the evolution of SARS-Co--2 since January 2020 and characterized Variants of Interest (VOIs) and Variants of Concern (VOCs) to guide comprehensive research. The changes can be monitored by monitoring changes in amino acid substitutions to inform countries about changes that may be needed to respond to the variant. Different countries may also report and designate other variants which are found in the patients. To contain the transmission through proven disease control measures and avoiding transmission to animal populations are important methods to decrease the chances of mutations having harmful health impacts. Research so far indicates that the general health and social measures and infection deterrence and management measures have been effective against COVID-19-related hospitalization and deaths. Table **1** summarizes the known variants of SARS-CoV-2.

Table 1. Known variants of SARS-CoV-2 [21].

WHO Label	Origin	Pango Lineage
Alpha	United Kingdom, September 2020	B.1.1.7
Beta	South Africa, May 2020	B.1.35.1
Gamma	Brazil, November 2020	P.1
Delta	India, November 2020	B.1.617.2
Omicron	Multiple countries, November 2021	B.1.1. 529

Structure and Activity Domain of SARS-CoV-2

SARS-CoV-2 is found to share a likeness with bat SARS-CoV. COVID-19 is a lineage B-beta-CoV related to SARS-like CoV, and RaTG13 originated in Yunnan, China, in 2013 [11]. It is an enveloped virus with an outer covering of fatty lipid molecules. The structure of COVID-19 and its mode of transmission is represented in (Fig. **1**) [22]. About 96% similarity in nucleotide sequencing suggested that SARS-CoV-2 might have emerged from a Bat SL-CoV. COVID-19 possesses the typical morphology of coronavirus [23]. 80% similarity has been obtained between the genome of COVID-19 with other human coronaviruses like SARS [24]. The spike glycoprotein of SARS-CoV-2 is the combination of bat SARS-CoV and Beta-CoV [25]. The life cycle of COVID-19 starts when the S protein gets attached to ACE2, which is the cellular receptor. Upon the binding, conformation changes take place in the S protein, which eases the entry of the virus within the cell membrane *via* an endosomal pathway. Inside the host cell, the RNA is released. Indian scientists have started working on genome sequencing of the virus to study the probability of mutation [26]. The transmission route is depicted in (Fig. **1**).

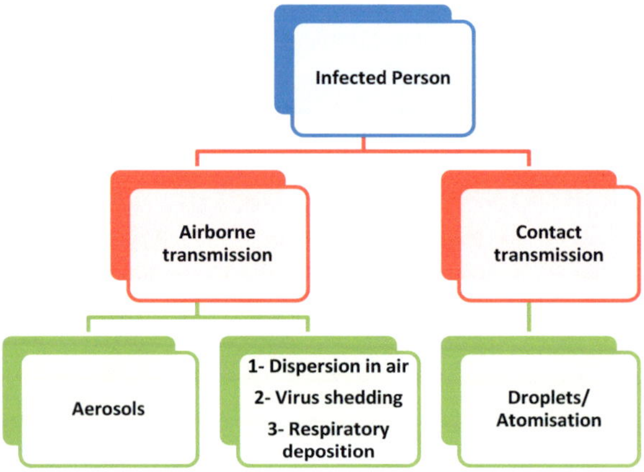

Fig. (1). COVID-19 transmission route.

The Search for Possible Medicinal Interventions

Guidelines and recommendations to facilitate infection control and methods to avert nosocomial spread are being issued [27]. The most effective treatment approach is to test the efficiency of the existing antiviral drugs. Antiviral drugs like ribavirin, interferon, lopinavir-ritonavir, *etc*., have been tested *in vitro* in previous betacoronavirus epidemics [28]. Remdesvir an adenosine analogue was also used previously against SARS and MERS-CoV [29]. *In vitro* testing of remdesivir is still going on to check its efficacy against SARS-CoV-2 [30]. Remdesivir was used against COVID-19 cases in the USA, and it was found that the clinical condition of the patients improved within one day [31]. Other probable drug candidates are chloroquine and camostatmesylate. Chloroquine, an anti-malarial drug, is known to block cell fusion in a virus and obstructs the glycosylation of the virus and ACE-2 receptors. It may also block cell entry of the pathogen. Camostat mesylate, also known as FOY 305, was primarily used to treat chronic pancreatitis and also found to inhibit the replication of SARS-CoV-2 [32]. Another effective therapy is the usage of recuperative plasma or serum of the recovered people developing antibody response which helps to neutralize the viral load. The ability of the virus to bind with the ACE-2 receptors may be explored to find out novel drugs. A receptor-binding domain (RBD) or a targeted antibody may block the binding of S protein and entry of the virus in host cells [33], but the strategy is time-bound and must be employed before the viral replication. Another way is to invent a molecule mimicking ACE-2, thereby blocking the S protein. The 2002 SARS incidence showed that soluble ACE-2 proteins inhibited the virus from cell invasion [34].

Mode of Spread

Conclusive pieces of evidence for the respiratory spread of SARS-CoV-2 have been given. Fomite transmission is also suspected, and sexual, faecal and bloodborne transmissions are hypothesized. Person-to-person transmission has also been identified as an important route. Contamination through the mucosa is also known [35]. The virus may be found in respiratory discharge, urine and stool [36]. The airborne spread was revealed in a community outbreak in Amoy Garden in HKSAR [37]. Research at the University of Nebraska Medical Centre disclosed the airborne nature of virus. Traces of the virus were found in the rooms and hallways where the patients were kept. Patients may create aerosols of the virus, posing a greater risk of transmission through personal items [38].

Respiratory Transmission

Respiratory transmission takes place when virus particles suspend on the aerosols exhaled by the infected person. Droplets can be particles larger than 5μm falling on the ground within approximately six feet, and aerosols lesser than 5 μm can remain suspended for a prolonged period [39]. Through aerosol, the virus can spread further. Proximity and closeness are important detriments of the risk associated with transmission [40]. Ventilation and its importance in curbing the spread are also pivotal, as opening windows allow better air movement [41].

Transmission through Direct Contact

Pieces of evidence of fomite transmission are circumstantial. Sharing elevators and restrooms may lead to fomite transmission [42]. Poor hand sanitization is also linked to elevated risk, and the use of chlorine and ethanol in households can decrease the risk [43].

Transmission through Domestic Pets

There is evidence showing that SARS-CoV-2 can infect domestic animals [44]. The virus can be transmitted between cats and ferrets through replication [45], although there is no evidence of transmission from domestic pets to humans.

Vertical Transmission

Reports suggest positive infection of SARS-CoV-2 IgM in neonates. IgM testing is also susceptible to false results. Reports also suggest nasopharyngeal positivity after delivery in the neonate [46].

Faecal–Oral (or Fecal Aerosol) Transmission

The faecal-oral route of spread was hypothesized after high concentrations of ACE-2 receptors were obtained in the small bowel [47]. The active virus has been infrequently obtained from faeces; however, viral RNA has been isolated from stool [48], leading to speculations about whether flushing can create virus aerosols and facilitate its transmission.

Clinical Symptoms with Special Emphasis on Respiratory Functionalities

COVID-19 is designated as a respiratory disease, with the infection reaching up to the lungs and travelling down the airways. The virus can affect the upper and lower respiratory tracts. In severe cases, the infection reaches the lungs filling them with fluid and debris. A person with already affected lungs may find it difficult to cope with the viral load. The incubation period for the virus ranges from one to fourteen days. Symptoms of Acute Respiratory Distress Syndrome (ARDS) are developed initially. Viral pneumonia is also common, causing respiratory damage in severe cases [49]. The improper lung functioning may be due to lung fibrosis and muscle weakness [50]. The survivors of the HKSAR outbreak showed impaired diffusion capacity of the lungs in 24% of the survivors [51]. A high concentration of cytokines has also been linked to disease severity [52].

AIR POLLUTION AS A CONTRIBUTING FACTOR

The spread of COVID-19 may be facilitated by ambient air pollution levels as air pollution is known to assist respiratory troubles. The virus, once inside the body, moves to the respiratory tract. A research study has declared that the death rate due to the diseases is associated with $PM_{2.5}$ levels. Countries with high particulate concentrations are more likely to have a high caseload [53]. The spread of the virus may be influenced by airborne particulate matter. China, where the virus originated, has high annual pollution levels, and in 2016, 4000 deaths were reported due to exposure to air pollution [53]. During the SARS outbreak in China during the year 2002, it was seen that the mortality rate was higher in regions with moderate air pollution index (API), and those exposed to high APIs were twice as susceptible to die as compared to those exposed to low APIs [54]. High particulate contamination may assist in the spread of the virus. Air pollutants with oxidizing nature lead to weak immune functions and impaired lung efficiency to clear off the virus. The positive change in the air quality during the lockdown phases may prove effective for the containment of the disease [55]. Particulate matter inflames and damages the lungs' lining, thereby hampering the body's response to fight respiratory infections. Children exposed to high particulate concentration may have malfunctioned lungs. Short-term exposure to high O_3 and PM_{10} concentrations has been linked to complaints of COPD and pneumonia and associated hospitalizations in elderly people, particularly during summer [56]. Regions like Lombardy and Emilia Romagna in Italy have reported high caseloads, and these regions also have high pollution levels. The virus may have long-range transportation as it can get adsorbed on the surface of particulate matter. A recent study has concluded that the virus can remain suspended for about thirty minutes in the air. Cigarette smoking is another factor linked with respiratory disorders and associated with higher DC-SIGN gene expression in the lungs of smokers and elderly people [57]. A study between1998-2015 revealed an annual increase of 1.7 million smokers in India, suggesting that the smoking rate in men doubled between 15-69 years and the habit was more prominent in the age group of 15-29 years [58]. They may be at a higher risk as their lungs might be already compromised. In another multi-centric study in India, COPD was found to be more prevalent in smokers in megacities like Delhi, Kanpur, Chandigarh and Bangalore [59]. The immunity of people living in cities with high pollution is already compromised. Air pollutants may stimulate oxidative stress in the airways leading to an inflammatory response and releasing inflammatory cells and mediators, harming the respiratory system [60]. (Fig. **2**) represents the likely spread of the virus through particulate matter.

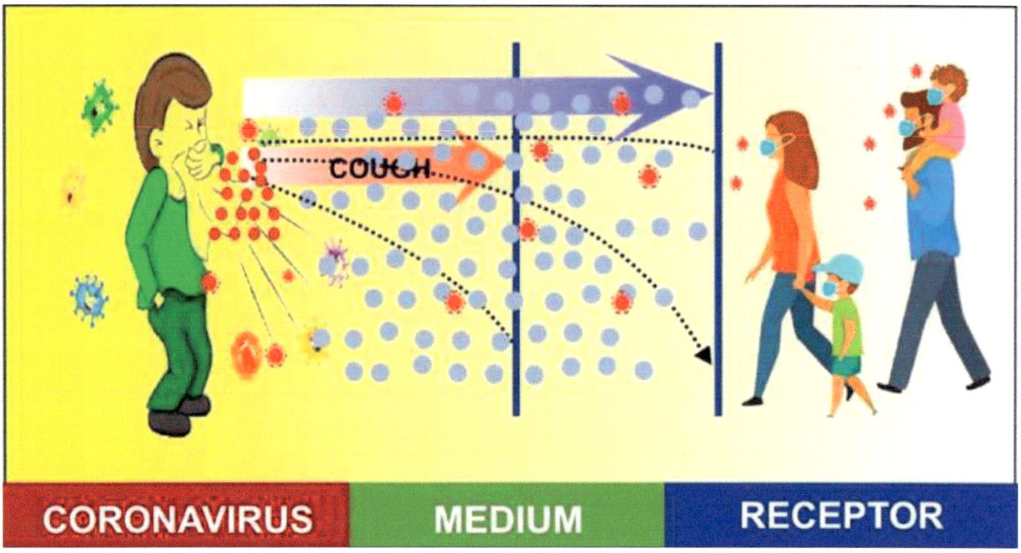

Fig. (2). The source, transmission and receptor cycle involving particulate matter.

Studies Suggesting an Alleged Association between Air Quality and COVID-19

A study conducted in 120 cities in China in the year 2020 took into account the concentrations of $PM_{2.5}$, PM_{10}, SO_2, CO, NO_2 and O_3 and weather conditions and the findings revealed that the concentration of these pollutants had an impact on the caseload. A 10-$\mu g/m^3$ hike in the concentration was linked with 2.24%, 1.76%, 6.94% and 4.76% hike in confirmed cases related to $PM_{2.5}$, PM_{10}, NO_2 and $O_{3,}$ pointing out a significant association of air pollution with COVID-19 cases [61]. Lombardy and Po Valley in Northern Italy, having high particulate concentration, witnessed a high number of cases, approximately about 80% of the total caseload [62]. Another study conducted in Germany, France, Italy and Spain also found that high concentrations of NO_2 impacted the death rate [63]. A study by the Harward School of Public Health has confirmed a link between Particulate concentration and COVID-19 mortality rate [64]. Particulate matter may absorb the virus on its surface leading to its spread. Recent findings have marked the presence of viral RNA on particulate matter. E gene was used as a molecular marker producing a positive result in 15 filters. The second clinical laboratory tested 34 RNA extractions for the E, N and RdRP genes, with 7 positive results [65]. The study is the first to provide concrete evidence of the SARS-CoV-2-RNA on ambient PM, suggesting that a high concentration of particulate matter could influence virus clustering by decreasing their diffusion coefficients, leading to the persistence of the virus for a longer period in the environment. The spike in air pollutants in ambient air might serve as a vector or carrier of COVID-19, facilitating its transmission farther. Table **2** summarizes some studies finding a relationship between air pollution and the COVID-19 caseload.

Table 2. Few reported studies showing a relation between air pollution and COVID-19 cases.

S.No.	Findings of the Study	Region	Reference
1	Levels of PM and NO_x map increased the number of COVID-19 infections in the UK Biobank.	England	https://doi.org/10.1016/j.envpol.2020.115859
2	Long-term air-quality data correlate with Covid-19 in the Italian provinces.	Italy	https://doi.org/10.1016/j.envpol.2020.114732
3	Positive associations of $PM_{2.5}$, PM_{10}, CO, NO_2 and O_3 with the COVID-19 caseload.	China	https://doi.org/10.1016/j.scitotenv.2020.138704
4	Artificial Neural Networks (ANNs) experiments have determined the concentration of $PM_{2.5}$ and PM_{10} linked to COVID-19-related deaths.	France	https://doi.org/10.1016/j.apenergy.2020.115835
5	Short-term exposure to suspended particles might have an association with respiratory infections caused by COVID-19.	Japan	https://doi.org/10.1016/j.envres.2020.110042
6	The daily $PM_{2.5}$ and PM_{10} concentrations and the daily CFR exhibited similarities concerning their temporal variation curves.	China	https://doi.org/10.1016/j.envres.2020.109941
7	1g/m^3 in $PM_{2.5}$ was linked with an 8% increase in the death rate.	USA	https://doi.org/10.1101/2020.04.05.20054502
8	The daily $PM_{2.5}$ and PM_{10} concentrations and the daily CFR exhibited similarity concerning their temporal variation curves.	China	https://doi.org/10.1016/j.envres.2020.109941
9	Increase the intensity of COVID-19 cases across all states except Massachusetts, associated with pollution levels.	USA	https://doi.org/10.1016/j.envres.2020.110189

(Table 2) cont.....

S.No.	Findings of the Study	Region	Reference
10	Air pollution assists in the spread of COVID-19 by carriers like $PM_{2.5}$, PM_{10} and by the pro-inflammatory effect of pollutants in the respiratory tract. Amazon fire and burns, air pollution in a zone like MANAUS.	Brazil	https://doi.org/10.7717/peerj.9322
11	$PM_{2.5}$ and NO_2 are responsible for COVID-19 deaths. Increasing levels of economic growth spur air pollution in New York state.	USA	https://doi.org/10.1016/j.jenvman.2021.112241
12	$PM_{2.5}$ and PM_{10} might be responsible for COVID-19 spread.	India	https://doi.org/10.1080/15275922.2020.1836082
13	Chronic exposure to $PM_{2.5}$, correlated with alveolar ACE-2 receptor over-expression. NO_2 concentration may lead to lung damage.	Italy	https://doi.org/10.1016/j.jinf.2020.05.031
14	AQI effect on the confirmed cases in the temperature range of 10–20 °C may be stronger. The impact of AQI on the spread of COVID-19 may be enhanced under low relative humidity.	China	https://doi.org/10.1016/j.scitotenv.2020.139211

Is Indoor Air Pollution Neglected Here?

According to WHO, ambient and household pollution causes the death of seven million people globally on an annual basis. Developing and under-developed nations are at high risk as the population is exposed to high indoor and outdoor pollutants [66]. We spend more than 80% of our time indoors, and exposure to household pollution accounts for 7.7% of global mortality [67]. People are not much aware of indoor air pollution. Pneumonia-related mortalities in children who are less than 5 years of age are caused by soot generated from the PM. Deaths from household air pollution are a leading cause of non-communicable diseases in developing and under-developed countries. Particulate matter is a pollutant of special concern, and smaller-sized particles ($PM_{2.5}$ or smaller) are usually more hazardous and detrimental to respiratory health. Indoor air pollutants can cause asthma, chronic bronchitis and cough, lung irritation, pneumonia and, most important, decreased resistance to respiratory infections [68].

Pathophysiology of SARS-CoV-2 and Similarity in Mechanistic Action with Particulate Matter

The reproduction of coronavirus starts from host living cells. The virus contains genetic material inside its protein envelope. Inside the host, the virus makes contact with the cells of the nose, throat or lungs. Through its spike, the virus gets inserted into the receptor molecule of the host cell membrane. This action facilitates the virus inside the host cell [69]. The human lungs have lobes. Normally, the air we breathe travels through the trachea or windpipe, bronchioles and eventually into the alveoli. Cilia having a hair-like structure continually push the mucus and germs out of the airways and drive them out by cough. The immune system shields against viruses and other pathogens that trespass the mucus and cilia, and enter the alveoli of the respiratory system. If the immune system is weakened then coronavirus overwhelms the host immune cells and bronchioles and alveoli become inflamed. The inflammation causes the host alveoli to fill with fluid, making it difficult for the host body to get the oxygen it needs. The further process of inflammation develops Lobar pneumonia, *i.e.*, one of the lobes of the lungs gets infected, or bronchopneumonia which affects many areas of the lungs. Particulate matter increases the chances of inflammation and increases both neutrophils and inflammatory cytokines in the lungs [70]. An increase in serum 8-isoprostane in broncho-alveolar lavage fluid or induced sputum also causes pneumonia in the body. The surface of $PM_{2.5}$ is enriched with Fe, Cu, Zn, Mn and other transition elements, polyaromatic Hydrocarbon, lipopolysaccharide, *etc*. The components facilitate the free radical generation in the lung, consume antioxidant ingredients and cause oxidative stress. If we compare the infection strategy of both particulate matter and COVID-19 infection, it is understood that both are involved in respiratory inflammation. Particulate matter as nano-scavenger enters through the windpipe and then to the bronchi and bronchioles, same as in the case of COVID-19. Both PM and coronavirus cause oxidative stress in the body which helps in enhancing the susceptibility and severity of respiratory infection.

Household Characteristics and their Impact

The household conditions and the surroundings may also influence the spread of the disease. Our previous study showed that the densely populated areas had closely built houses, with inadequate ventilation and narrow parking spaces and were mostly surrounded by commercial markets, whereas the houses which were built along the roadside were situated adjacent to highways, experiencing heavy traffic flow all day. Building ventilation may help improve the air quality and minimize health issues, including the avoidance of COVID-19 transmission indoors. The physiopathology of the viral infection and the main cause of death include aggravated inflammation, particularly in the lungs, resulting in weakened pulmonary oxygen exchange and severe pneumonia. Congested houses with inadequate ventilation may also have low UV index and exposure to sunshine. It has been observed that the faster spread of COVID-19 is facilitated by low UV index and vitamin D levels [71]. The transmission is predominantly more effective in close, crowded, cramped indoor settings with scanty ventilation [72]. Ensuring proper ventilation may lower the risk of infection [73]. The importance of good indoor practices and ventilation is slowly coming to notice, and the Indian government issued guidelines on 26th April 2021 and instructed the people to wear masks even at home and avoid areas with poor ventilation. Consequently, besides the probable mode of action of airborne spread, other mechanisms of transmission in humans should be measured for a thorough interpretation of the impact of air quality on the virus spread.

Improvement in Air Quality during the Lockdown: Exploring the Positive Aspect of the Pandemic

Based on satellite measurements, several studies [74 - 77] have recently shown how air pollution has fallen dramatically in cities across the world due to lockdown measures enacted during COVID-19. Ground-level measurements confirm these observations. The lockdown orders associated with COVID-19 have had a profound impact on our atmospheric environment. With the reduction in industrial activities and residential automobile activity, the ambient concentrations of PM, CO, NO_2, and, in some cases, SO_2 were much lower than they normally are, likely due to a combination of lower emissions and meteorological conditions. In contrast to this, O_3 concentrations were higher than normal due to the reduction in emissions from traffic. The increase in O_3 concentrations can likely be attributed to a reduction in NO emissions, which thus reduces the reaction of NO with O_3 to form NO_2.

A study conducted in India observed a decrease of 43% and 31%, respectively, in the concentrations of particulate contamination [78]. In 2017, the National Council of Medical Research (ICMR) announced a community health emergency in the National capital Region (NCR) of Delhi owing to the increasing air pollution. Moreover, a pre and post-lockdown study conducted in Delhi showed a significant decrease in the concentrations of PM_{10}, $PM_{2.5}$, SO_2, NO_2, CO, O_3 and NH_3. PM_{10} and $PM_{2.5}$ reduced by half during the lockdown as compared to 2019 data of the same period [79]. Similarly, a recent air quality analysis conducted in prominent cities of the world, including New York, Los Angeles, Rome, Delhi, Mumbai, Beijing and Shanghai, showed a reduction in the concentration of $PM_{2.5}$ during lockdown [79].

Lucknow, a megacity located in North India, is on the WHO list of most polluted cities [80]. According to the latest WHO World Air 2019 report, Lucknow was placed in tenth position for high particulate concentration around the year. A comparison in the Air Quality Index concerning $PM_{2.5}$ in the Lucknow region is summarized in Table **3**. The AQI values have been obtained from the real-time monitoring stations in the city. The data depicts a very distinct and positive change in the air quality of Lucknow city. The improvement in the air quality may, in part, be responsible for the remarkable recovery rate of COVID-19 patients in the city.

Contribution of Meteorological Parameters

Strains like MERS-CoV, TEGV and MHV have shown decreased activity at higher temperatures viz 30-40 ^{0}C [81]. However, at lower temperatures up to 4 ^{0}C, the persistence can be as long as 28 days. At room temperature, HCoV-229E growth was more pronounced at 50% humidity. Meteorological parameters like temperature and humidity influenced the spread of SARS. A study conducted in Wuhan, China, to study the linkage between COVID-19 deaths and weather conditions, established an association between temperature and relative humidity with mortality. A positive association was established between diurnal temperature and mortality, but an inverse relationship was observed for relative humidity, suggesting that temperature and humidity are important parameters linked to COVID-19 mortality. During the study, the temperature ranged between 1.8 °C-18.7 ^{0}C, and the diurnal temperature ranged between 2 ^{0}C-17.5 ^{0}C [82]. A study conducted in Iran has analyzed the influence of ambient temperature and population size on the transmission of the virus. The sensibility of the ambient temperature and the sensitivity of the population size were investigated in different provinces of Iran, and it was found that ambient temperature had a linear relationship with the number of cases [83].

Table 3. Comparative AQI Data Concerning $PM_{2.5}$ in Lucknow city.

Comparative AQI Data Concerning $PM_{2.5}$ at Industrial Site							
April	2016	2017	2018	2019	2020	Difference with Max.	%Difference
1st Week	186±13	185±18	170±13	265±48	122±9	-143	117%
2nd Week	189±12	191±27	149±17	176±25	109±26	-82	75%
3rd Week	195±8	191±19	191±19	170±17	133±35	-62	46%
4th Week	191±5	239±51	192±24	217±27	105±23	-134	127%
4th Week	191±5	239±51	192±24	217±27	105±23	-134	127%
Comparative AQI Data Concerning $PM_{2.5}$ at Commercial Site							
April	2016	2017	2018	2019	2020	Difference with Max.	%Difference
1st Week	170±15	172±15	165±19	173±20	133±7	-40	30%
2nd Week	181±16	165±20	157±24	171±16	136±23	-45	33%

(Table 3) cont.....

Comparative AQI Data Concerning $PM_{2.5}$ at Industrial Site							
3rd Week	195±13	203±32	216±35	159±39	121±37	-95	79%
4th Week	173±12	212±28	209±40	213±38	125±30	-88	70%
Comparative AQI Data concerning $PM_{2.5}$ at Residential Site							
April	2016	2017	2018	2019	2020	Difference with Max.	%Difference
1st Week	171±20	184±13	146±24	176±46	84±21	-100	119%
2nd Week	177±7	179±30	132±20	142±24	102±22	-77	75%
3rd Week	177±10	186±24	182±11	130±30	105±17	-81	77%
4th Week	172±8	201±21	182±18	186±18	110±18	-91	83%

Natural Resources as Immunity Boosters- A Probable Preventive Measure

Strengthening the human immune system against the external undesirable responses can be attained by following a healthy dietary regime. The exploration of the diet with good health needs acceptance in daily life [84]. Low intake of fruits, vegetables, and whole grains can deprive the body of carotenoids, Vitamin D, E, flavonoids and omega-3 fatty acids, causing low immunity to air pollution and microbial infections [84]. Naturally, derived compounds have emerged as worthy therapeutic alternatives against several diseases and viral infections. The U.S. Food and Drug Administration (FDA) has approved 49% of small molecules, which were either natural products or their derivatives [85].

The probable role of herbal medicines and products has also been explored to fight against coronavirus infection [86]. Spices and herbs have high antioxidant and antimicrobial potential. They are rich sources of flavonoids, alkaloids, phenolic compounds, tannins, phenolic diterpenes, *etc* [86]. The traditional medicinal system is very popular in India, which has six systems of medicine, namely Ayurveda, yoga, Unani, Siddha, naturopathy, and homeopathy [87]. Ayurveda, the science of life, is a wholesome medical system. In India, around 20,000 plant species have been identified as having medicinal properties [88]. The antioxidant potential may improve respiratory functioning and reduce oxidative stress and inflammation. The mechanistic action includes boosting and functioning of the immune system, activation and containment of immune specialized cells, causing hindrance in several pathways, eventually leading to better immune responses and defence. At the onset of the viral infection, a "cytokine storm" in the body is generated, causing overexpression of immune cells and their cytokines, which, in a flu infection, is mostly linked with a rush of activated immune cells in the lungs [89]. There is an urgent and worldwide need to explore medicinal agents that can act against the virus as a precautionary measure and improve immunity. Table **4** lists some of the known immunity-boosting herbs and spices and their details.

Table 4. Few common spices and herbs of medicinal importance

S.No.	Herb/Spice	Common Name	Family	Phytoconstituents	Physiological Role
1	*Curcuma longa L.*	Turmeric	Zingiberaceae	Curcuminoids, steroids, polyphenols	Anti-inflammatory, anti-neoplastic, anti-angiogenic
2	*Zingiber officinale*	Ginger	Zingiberaceae	Zingiberol, paradol, shagols, zingerone	Antiemetic, antipyretic, analgesic, antiarthritic, antiinflamamtory
3	*Cinnamomum cassia*	Cinnamon	Lauraceae	(E)-cinnamaldehyde, (Z)-cinnamaldehyde β-caryophyllene, coumarin and α-ylangene	Antimicrobial, antiviral, antioxidant, antidiabetic, antihypertensive
4	*Syzgium aromaticum*	Clove	Myrtaceae	Flavanoids, hidroxicinamic acid, hidroxiphenylpropens, eugenol	Antimicrobial, antiemetic, carminative
5	*Piper nigrum*	Black pepper	Piperaceae	Piperine	Anti-inflammatory, anti-oxidant, antimicrobial, analgesic, antidepressant
6	*Ocimum basilicum*	Basil	Labiatae	Linalool, myrcene, carvone, fenchone, caryophyllene, farnesol	Antiviral
7	*Allium sativum L.*	Garlic	Liliaceae	Allicin, Methyl aalyl thiosulfanata	Anthelmintics, anti-inflammatory, antioxidant, antifungal
8	*Azadirachta indica*	Neem	Meliaceae	Nimbin, nimbidin, limonoids, nimbione, margocin	Insecticidal, antimicrobial, larvicidal, antimalarial, antibacterial
9	*Tinospora cordifolia*	Giloy	Ispermaceae	Berberine, b-sitosterol, coline, octacosanol, tetrahydropalmatine	Antidiabetic, anti-inflammatory, antiviral

CONCLUSION

The pieces of evidence so far suggest that COVID-19 is a respiratory disease that leads to severe ARDS and pneumonia. Mostly the spread is respiratory, and the virus suspends either on droplets or aerosols. The studies are establishing a correlation between COVID-19 and air pollution, particularly particulate matter, but at the same time, it is imperative to study the mechanism explaining the correlation. Nonetheless, both long-term and short-term exposures to high concentrations of pollutants are correlated to an increase in caseload related to COVID-19. Special care is necessary for people exposed to poor-quality air, making them more vulnerable to the infection as their lungs are already compromised. This broader environmental dimension has not been considered systematically, however, air pollution, exposure to bad air quality, long-term absorption of emissions and particulate matter, or breathing of CO_2 through cooking stoves exposure and other forms of emission need to be addressed as well in context to spread of infection, especially in India as of the world's top 30 most polluted cities during 2019, 21 belong to India. This factor will be crucial in the coming time for the spread of the infection. Not only ambient pollution, indoor settings, proximity and ventilation practices may also govern the transmission dynamics and must be thoroughly explored.

CONSENT FOR PUBLICATION

Not applicable.

CONFLICT OF INTEREST

The authors declare no conflict of interest, financial or otherwise.

ACKNOWLEDGEMENT

None declared.

REFERENCES

[1] Drosten C, Günther S, Preiser W, *et al.* Identification of a novel coronavirus in patients with severe acute respiratory syndrome. N Engl J Med 2003; 348(20): 1967-76. [http://dx.doi.org/10.1056/NEJMoa030747] [PMID: 12690091]

[2] Desforges M, Le Coupanec A, Brison É, Meessen-Pinard M, Talbot PJ. Neuroinvasive and neurotropic human respiratory coronaviruses: potential neurovirulent agents in humans. Adv Exp Med Biol 2014; 807: 75-96. [http://dx.doi.org/10.1007/978-81-322-1777-0_6] [PMID: 24619619]

[3] Tajima M. Morphology of transmissible gastroenteritis virus of pigs. Arch Virol 1970; 29(1): 105-8. [http://dx.doi.org/10.1007/BF01253886] [PMID: 4195092]

[4] Chin AWH, Chu JTS, Perera MRA, *et al.* Stability of SARS-CoV-2 in different environmental conditions Lancet Microb. 2020; 1-e10. [http://dx.doi.org/10.1016/S2666-5247(20)30003-3]

[5] Meyerowitz EA, Richterman A, Gandhi RT, Sax PE. Transmission of SARS-CoV-2: A Review of Viral, Host, and Environmental Factors. Ann Intern Med 2021; 174(1): 69-79. [http://dx.doi.org/10.7326/M20-5008] [PMID: 32941052]

[6] Hoffmann M, Kleine-Weber H, Schroeder S, *et al.* SARS-CoV-2 cell entry depends on ACE2 and TMPRSS2 and is blocked by a clinically proven protease inhibitor. Cell 2020; 181(2): 271-280.e8. [http://dx.doi.org/10.1016/j.cell.2020.02.052] [PMID: 32142651]

[7] Jing QL, Liu MJ, Zhang ZB, *et al.* Household secondary attack rate of COVID-19 and associated determinants in Guangzhou, China: a retrospective cohort study. Lancet Infect Dis 2020; 20(10): 1141-50.
[http://dx.doi.org/10.1016/S1473-3099(20)30471-0] [PMID: 32562601]

[8] Gudbjartsson DF, Helgason A, Jonsson H, *et al.* Spread of SARSCoV-2 in the Icelandic population. N Engl J Med 2020; 382(24): 2302-15.
[http://dx.doi.org/10.1056/NEJMoa2006100] [PMID: 32289214]

[9] Bunyavanich S, Do A, Vicencio A. Nasal gene expression of angiotensin-converting enzyme 2 in children and adults. JAMA 2020; 323(23): 2427-9.
[http://dx.doi.org/10.1001/jama.2020.8707] [PMID: 32432657]

[10] Chen H, Guo J, Wang C, *et al.* Clinical characteristics and intrauterine vertical transmission potential of COVID-19 infection in nine pregnant women: a retrospective review of medical records. Lancet 2020; 395(10226): 809-15.
[http://dx.doi.org/10.1016/S0140-6736(20)30360-3] [PMID: 32151335]

[11] Fan Y, Zhao K, Shi ZL, Zhou P. Bat Coronaviruses in China. Viruses 2019; 11(3): 210.
[http://dx.doi.org/10.3390/v11030210] [PMID: 30832341]

[12] 2020.https://www.greencarcongress.com/2020/03/20200317-epha.html

[13] Cheng VCC, Lau SKP, Woo PCY, Yuen KY. Severe acute respiratory syndrome coronavirus as an agent of emerging and reemerging infection. Clin Microbiol Rev 2007; 20(4): 660-94.
[http://dx.doi.org/10.1128/CMR.00023-07] [PMID: 17934078]

[14] Mesel-Lemoine M, Millet J, Vidalain PO, *et al.* A human coronavirus responsible for the common cold massively kills dendritic cells but not monocytes. J Virol 2012; 86(14): 7577-87.
[http://dx.doi.org/10.1128/JVI.00269-12] [PMID: 22553325]

[15] Abebe EC, Dejenie TA, Shiferaw MY, *et al.* The newly emerged COVID-19 disease: a systemic review. Virol J 17 2020; 17: 96.

[16] Mann R, Perisetti A, Gajendran M, Gandhi Z, Umapathy C, Goyal H. Clinical Characteristics, Diagnosis, and Treatment of Major Coronavirus Outbreaks. Front Med (Lausanne) 2020; 7: 581521.
[http://dx.doi.org/10.3389/fmed.2020.581521] [PMID: 33282890]

[17] Webster RG. Wet markets—a continuing source of severe acute respiratory syndrome and influenza? Lancet 2004; 363(9404): 234-6.
[http://dx.doi.org/10.1016/S0140-6736(03)15329-9] [PMID: 14738798]

[18] Cui J, Li F, Shi ZL. Origin and evolution of pathogenic coronaviruses. Nat Rev Microbiol 2019; 17(3): 181-92.
[http://dx.doi.org/10.1038/s41579-018-0118-9] [PMID: 30531947]

[19] Ksiazek TG, Erdman D, Goldsmith CS, *et al.* A novel coronavirus associated with severe acute respiratory syndrome. N Engl J Med 2003; 348(20): 1953-66.
[http://dx.doi.org/10.1056/NEJMoa030781] [PMID: 12690092]

[20] Andersen KG, Rambaut A, Lipkin WI, Holmes EC, Garry RF. The proximal origin of SARS-CoV-2. Nat Med 2020; 26(4): 450-2.
[http://dx.doi.org/10.1038/s41591-020-0820-9] [PMID: 32284615]

[21] Otter JA, Donskey C, Yezli S, Douthwaite S, Goldenberg SD, Weber DJ. Transmission of SARS and MERS coronaviruses and influenza virus in healthcare settings: the possible role of dry surface contamination. J Hosp Infect 2016; 92(3): 235-50.
[http://dx.doi.org/10.1016/j.jhin.2015.08.027] [PMID: 26597631]

[22] Zhou P, Yang XL, Wang XG, *et al.* A pneumonia outbreak associated with a new coronavirus of probable bat origin. Nature 2020; 579(7798): 270-3.
[http://dx.doi.org/10.1038/s41586-020-2012-7] [PMID: 32015507]

[23] Shereen MA, Khan S, Kazmi A, Bashir N, Siddique R. COVID-19 infection: Emergence, transmission, and characteristics of human coronaviruses. J Adv Res 2020; 24: 91-8. [http://dx.doi.org/10.1016/j.jare.2020.03.005] [PMID: 32257431]

[24] Wu F, Zhao S, Yu B, *et al.* A new coronavirus associated with human respiratory disease in China. Nature 2020; 579(7798): 265-9. [http://dx.doi.org/10.1038/s41586-020-2008-3] [PMID: 32015508]

[25] Li B, Si HR, Zhu Y, *et al.* Discovery of Bat Coronaviruses through Surveillance and Probe Capture-Based Next-Generation Sequencing. MSphere 2020; 5(1): e00807-19. [http://dx.doi.org/10.1128/mSphere.00807-19] [PMID: 31996413]

[26] Raoult D, Zumla A, Locatelli F, Ippolito G, Kroemer G. Coronavirus infections: Epidemiological, clinical and immunological features and hypotheses. Cell Stress 2020; 4(4): 66-75. [http://dx.doi.org/10.15698/cst2020.04.216] [PMID: 32292881]

[27] Wax RS, Christian MD. Practical recommendations for critical care and anesthesiology teams caring for novel coronavirus (2019-nCoV) patients. Can J Anaesth 2020; 67(5): 568-76. [http://dx.doi.org/10.1007/s12630-020-01591-x] [PMID: 32052373]

[28] Chu CM, Cheng VC, Hung IF, *et al.* Role of lopinavir/ritonavir in the treatment of SARS: initial virological and clinical findings. Thorax 2004; 59(3): 252-6. [http://dx.doi.org/10.1136/thorax.2003.012658] [PMID: 14985565]

[29] Sheahan TP, Sims AC, Graham RL, *et al.* Broad-spectrum antiviral GS-5734 inhibits both epidemic and zoonotic coronaviruses. Sci Transl Med 2017; 9(396): eaal3653. [http://dx.doi.org/10.1126/scitranslmed.aal3653] [PMID: 28659436]

[30] Wang M, Cao R, Zhang L, *et al.* Remdesivir and chloroquine effectively inhibit the recently emerged novel coronavirus (2019-nCoV) *in vitro*. Cell Res 2020; 30(3): 269-71. [http://dx.doi.org/10.1038/s41422-020-0282-0] [PMID: 32020029]

[31] Holshue ML, DeBolt C, Lindquist S, *et al.* First Case of 2019 Novel Coronavirus in the United States. N Engl J Med 2020; 382(10): 929-36. [http://dx.doi.org/10.1056/NEJMoa2001191] [PMID: 32004427]

[32] Yamawaki H, Futagami S, Kaneko K, *et al.* Camostat Mesilate, Pancrelipase, and Rabeprazole Combination Therapy Improves Epigastric Pain in Early Chronic Pancreatitis and Functional Dyspepsia with Pancreatic Enzyme Abnormalities. Digestion 2019; 99(4): 283-92. [http://dx.doi.org/10.1159/000492813] [PMID: 30391941]

[33] Li W, Moore MJ, Vasilieva N, *et al.* Angiotensin-converting enzyme 2 is a functional receptor for the SARS coronavirus. Nature 2003; 426(6965): 450-4. [http://dx.doi.org/10.1038/nature02145] [PMID: 14647384]

[34] Moore MJ, Dorfman T, Li W, *et al.* Retroviruses pseudotyped with the severe acute respiratory syndrome coronavirus spike protein efficiently infect cells expressing angiotensin-converting enzyme 2. J Virol 2004; 78(19): 10628-35. [http://dx.doi.org/10.1128/JVI.78.19.10628-10635.2004] [PMID: 15367630]

[35] Shao PL, Hsueh PR, Chang LY, *et al.* Development of immunoglobulin G enzyme-linked immunosorbent assay for the serodiagnosis of severe acute respiratory syndrome. J Biomed Sci 2005; 12(1): 59-64. [http://dx.doi.org/10.1007/s11373-004-8184-6] [PMID: 15864739]

[36] Loon S-C, Teoh SCB, Oon LLE, *et al.* The severe acute respiratory syndrome coronavirus in tears. Br J Ophthalmol 2004; 88(7): 861-3. [http://dx.doi.org/10.1136/bjo.2003.035931] [PMID: 15205225]

[37] Yu ITS, Li Y, Wong TW, *et al.* Evidence of airborne transmission of the severe acute respiratory syndrome virus. N Engl J Med 2004; 350(17): 1731-9. [http://dx.doi.org/10.1056/NEJMoa032867] [PMID: 15102999]

[38] Ijaz MK, Brunner AH, Sattar SA, Nair RC, Johnson-Lussenburg CM. Survival characteristics of airborne human coronavirus 229E. J Gen Virol 1985; 66(12): 2743-8. [http://dx.doi.org/10.1099/0022-1317-66-12-2743] [PMID: 2999318]

[39] Wei J, Li Y. Airborne spread of infectious agents in the indoor environment. Am J Infect Control 2016; 44(9) (Suppl.): S102-8. [http://dx.doi.org/10.1016/j.ajic.2016.06.003] [PMID: 27590694]

[40] Courtemanche C, Garuccio J, Le A, Pinkston J, Yelowitz A. Strong social distancing measures in the United States reduced the COVID-19 growth rate. Health Aff (Millwood) 2020; 39(7): 1237-46. [http://dx.doi.org/10.1377/hlthaff.2020.00608] [PMID: 32407171]

[41] Wang Y, Tian H, Zhang L, *et al.* Reduction of secondary transmission of SARS-CoV-2 in households by face mask use, disinfection and social distancing: a cohort study in Beijing, China. BMJ Glob Health 2020; 5(5): e002794. [http://dx.doi.org/10.1136/bmjgh-2020-002794] [PMID: 32467353]

[42] Cai J, Sun W, Huang J, Gamber M, Wu J, He G. Indirect virus transmission in cluster of COVID-19 cases, Wenzhou, China, 2020. Emerg Infect Dis 2020; 26(6): 1343-5. [http://dx.doi.org/10.3201/eid2606.200412] [PMID: 32163030]

[43] Tian H, Liu Y, Li Y, *et al.* An investigation of transmission control measures during the first 50 days of the COVID-19 epidemic in China. Science 2020; 368(6491): 638-42. [http://dx.doi.org/10.1126/science.abb6105] [PMID: 32234804]

[44] Shi J, Wen Z, Zhong G, *et al.* Susceptibility of ferrets, cats, dogs, and other domesticated animals to SARS–coronavirus 2. Science 2020; 368(6494): 1016-20. [http://dx.doi.org/10.1126/science.abb7015] [PMID: 32269068]

[45] Richard M, Kok A, de Meulder D, *et al.* SARS-CoV-2 is transmitted *via* contact and *via* the air between ferrets. Nat Commun 2020; 11(1): 3496. [http://dx.doi.org/10.1038/s41467-020-17367-2] [PMID: 32641684]

[46] Zeng L, Xia S, Yuan W, *et al.* Neonatal early-onset infection with SARS-CoV-2 in 33 neonates born to mothers with COVID-19 in Wuhan, China. JAMA Pediatr 2020; 174(7): 722-5. [http://dx.doi.org/10.1001/jamapediatrics.2020.0878] [PMID: 32215598]

[47] Gu J, Han B, Wang J. COVID-19: gastrointestinal manifestations and potential fecal-oral transmission. Gastroenterology 2020; 158(6): 1518-9. [http://dx.doi.org/10.1053/j.gastro.2020.02.054] [PMID: 32142785]

[48] Wang W, Xu Y, Gao R, *et al.* Detection of SARS-CoV-2 in Different Types of Clinical Specimens. JAMA 2020; 323(18): 1843-4. [http://dx.doi.org/10.1001/jama.2020.3786] [PMID: 32159775]

[49] Booth CM, Matukas LM, Tomlinson GA, *et al.* Clinical features and short-term outcomes of 144 patients with SARS in the greater Toronto area. JAMA 2003; 289(21): 2801-9. [http://dx.doi.org/10.1001/jama.289.21.JOC30885] [PMID: 12734147]

[50] Yudin MH, Steele DM, Sgro MD, Read SE, Kopplin P, Gough KA. Severe acute respiratory syndrome in pregnancy. Obstet Gynecol 2005; 105(1): 124-7. [http://dx.doi.org/10.1097/01.AOG.0000151598.49129.de] [PMID: 15625153]

[51] Ong K-C, Ng AW, Lee LS, *et al.* Pulmonary function and exercise capacity in survivors of severe acute respiratory syndrome. Eur Respir J 2004; 24(3): 436-42. [http://dx.doi.org/10.1183/09031936.04.00007104] [PMID: 15358703]

[52] Hui DS, Wong KT, Ko FW, *et al.* The 1-year impact of severe acute respiratory syndrome on pulmonary function, exercise capacity, and quality of life in a cohort of survivors. Chest 2005; 128(4): 2247-61. [http://dx.doi.org/10.1378/chest.128.4.2247] [PMID: 16236881]

[53] He L, Zhang S, Hu J, *et al.* On-road emission measurements of reactive nitrogen compounds from heavy-duty diesel trucks in China. Environ Pollut 2020; 262: 114280. [http://dx.doi.org/10.1016/j.envpol.2020.114280] [PMID: 32146368]

[54] Cui Y, Zhang Z-F, Froines J, *et al.* Air pollution and case fatality of SARS in the People's Republic of China: an ecologic study. Env Hea: A Global Acc Sci Sou 2003; 20(2): 15. [http://dx.doi.org/10.1186/1476-069X-2-15]

[55] Dutheil F, Baker JS, Navel V. COVID-19 as a factor influencing air pollution. Environ Pollut 2020; 263(Pt A): 114466. [http://dx.doi.org/10.1016/j.envpol.2020.114466]

[56] Medina-Ramón M, Zanobetti A, Schwartz J. The effect of ozone and PM10 on hospital admissions for pneumonia and chronic obstructive pulmonary disease: a national multicity study. Am J Epidemiol 2006; 163(6): 579-88. [http://dx.doi.org/10.1093/aje/kwj078] [PMID: 16443803]

[57] Chan JF-W, Yuan S, Kok K-H, *et al.* A familial cluster of pneumonia associated with the 2019 novel coronavirus indicating person-to-person transmission: a study of a family cluster. Lancet 2020. S0140-6736(20):30154-9. [http://dx.doi.org/10.1016/S0140-6736(20)30154-9]

[58] Mishra S, Joseph RA, Gupta PC, *et al.* Trends in bidi and cigarette smoking in India from 1998 to 2015, by age, gender and education. BMJ Glob Health 2016; 1(1): e000005. [http://dx.doi.org/10.1136/bmjgh-2015-000005] [PMID: 28588906]

[59] Jindal SK, Aggarwal AN, Chaudhry K, *et al.* A multicentric study on epidemiology of chronic obstructive pulmonary disease and its relationship with tobacco smoking and environmental tobacco smoke exposure. Indian J Chest Dis Allied Sci 2006; 48(1): 23-9. [PMID: 16482948]

[60] de Souza A, Guo Y, Pavão H, *et al.* Effects of Air Pollution on Disease Respiratory. Structures Lag Health 2014; 6: 1333-9.

[61] Corman VM, Landt O, Kaiser M, *et al.* Detection of 2019 novel coronavirus (2019-nCoV) by real-time RT-PCR. Euro Surveill 2020; 25(3): 2000045. [http://dx.doi.org/10.2807/1560-7917.ES.2020.25.3.2000045] [PMID: 31992387]

[62] Dettori M, Deiana G, Balletto G, *et al.* Air pollutants and risk of death due to COVID-19 in Italy. Environ Res 2021; 192: 110459. [http://dx.doi.org/10.1016/j.envres.2020.110459] [PMID: 33188767]

[63] Villeneuve PJ, Goldberg MS. Methodological Considerations for Epidemiological Studies of Air Pollution and the SARS and COVID-19 Coronavirus Outbreaks. Environ Health Perspect 2020; 128(9): 095001. [http://dx.doi.org/10.1289/EHP7411] [PMID: 32902328]

[64] Zhang R, Li Y, Zhang AL, Wang Y, Molina MJ. Identifying airborne transmission as the dominant route for the spread of COVID-19. Proc Natl Acad Sci USA 2020; 117(26): 14857-63. [http://dx.doi.org/10.1073/pnas.2009637117] [PMID: 32527856]

[65] Setti L, Passarini F, De Gennaro G, *et al.* SARS-Cov-2RNA found on particulate matter of Bergamo in Northern Italy: First evidence. Environ Res 2020; 188: 109754. [http://dx.doi.org/10.1016/j.envres.2020.109754] [PMID: 32526492]

[66] Anenberg SC, Achakulwisut P, Brauer M, Moran D, Apte JS, Henze DK. Particulate matter-attributable mortality and relationships with carbon dioxide in 250 urban areas worldwide. Sci Rep 2019; 9(1): 11552. [http://dx.doi.org/10.1038/s41598-019-48057-9] [PMID: 31399636]

[67] Hadley MB, Vedanthan R, Fuster V. Air pollution and cardiovascular disease: a window of opportunity. Nat Rev Cardiol 2018; 15(4): 193-4.

[http://dx.doi.org/10.1038/nrcardio.2017.207] [PMID: 29297510]

[68] Raj K. Air pollution and respiratory health. J Adv Pediatr Child Health 2020; 3(1): 032-7. [http://dx.doi.org/10.29328/journal.japch.1001015]

[69] Sanità di Toppi L, Sanità di Toppi L, Bellini E. Novel Coronavirus: How Atmospheric Particulate Affects Our Environment and Health. Challenges 2020; 11(1): 6. [http://dx.doi.org/10.3390/challe11010006]

[70] Xing YF, Xu YH, Shi MH, Lian YX. The impact of $PM_{2.5}$ on the human respiratory system. J Thorac Dis 2016; 8(1): E69-74. [PMID: 26904255]

[71] Benskin LL. A Basic Review of the Preliminary Evidence That COVID-19 Risk and Severity Is Increased in Vitamin D Deficiency. Front Public Health 2020; 8: 513. [http://dx.doi.org/10.3389/fpubh.2020.00513] [PMID: 33014983]

[72] Zimmerman T, Siddiqui SA, Bischoff W, Ibrahim SA. Tackling Airborne Virus Threats in the Food Industry: A Proactive Approach. Int J Environ Res Public Health 2021; 18(8): 4335. [http://dx.doi.org/10.3390/ijerph18084335] [PMID: 33921880]

[73] Dai H, Zhao B. Association of the infection probability of COVID-19 with ventilation rates in confined spaces. Build Simul 2020; 13(6): 1321-7. [http://dx.doi.org/10.1007/s12273-020-0703-5] [PMID: 32837691]

[74] Bray CD, Nahas A, Battye WH, Aneja VP. Impact of lockdown during the COVID-19 outbreak on multi-scale air quality. Atmos Environ 2021; 254: 118386. [http://dx.doi.org/10.1016/j.atmosenv.2021.118386] [PMID: 33841025]

[75] Shi X, Brasseur GP. The response in air quality to the reduction of Chinese economic activities during the COVID-19 outbreak, Geophys. Res Lett 2020; 47 Article e2020GL088070.

[76] Venter ZS, Aunan K, Chowdhury S, Lelieveld J. COVID-19 lockdowns cause global air pollution declines. Proc Natl Acad Sci USA 2020; 117(32): 18984-90. [http://dx.doi.org/10.1073/pnas.2006853117] [PMID: 32723816]

[77] Bauwens M, Compernolle S, Stavrakou T, *et al.* Impact of Coronavirus Outbreak on NO2 Pollution Assessed Using TROPOMI and OMI Observations. American Geophysical Union 2020. [http://dx.doi.org/10.1029/2020GL087978]

[78] Nakada LYK, Urban RC. COVID-19 pandemic: Impacts on the air quality during the partial lockdown in São Paulo state, Brazil. Sci Total Environ 2020; 730: 139087. [http://dx.doi.org/10.1016/j.scitotenv.2020.139087] [PMID: 32380370]

[79] Chauhan A, Singh RP. Decline in $PM_{2.5}$ concentrations over major cities around the world associated with COVID-19. Environ Res 2020; 187: 109634. [http://dx.doi.org/10.1016/j.envres.2020.109634] [PMID: 32416359]

[80] Lawrence AJ, Khan T, Azad I. Indoor Air Quality Assessment and Health Impact in context to Household conditions in Lucknow. Glob NEST J 2019; 22(1): 28-41.

[81] Avendano M, Derkach P, Swan S. Clinical course and management of SARS in health care workers in Toronto: a case series. CMAJ 2003; 168(13): 1649-60. [PMID: 12821618]

[82] Ma Y, Zhao Y, Liu J, *et al.* Effects of temperature variation and humidity on the death of COVID-19 in Wuhan, China. Sci Total Environ 2020; 724: 138226. [http://dx.doi.org/10.1016/j.scitotenv.2020.138226] [PMID: 32408453]

[83] Jahangiri M, Jahangiri M, Najafgholipour M. The sensitivity and specificity analyses of ambient temperature and population size on the transmission rate of the novel coronavirus (COVID-19) in different provinces of Iran. Sci Total Environ 2020; 728: 138872. [http://dx.doi.org/10.1016/j.scitotenv.2020.138872] [PMID: 32335407]

[84] Sultan MT, Buttxs MS, Qayyum MMN, Suleria HAR. Immunity: plants as effective mediators. Crit Rev Food Sci Nutr 2014; 54(10): 1298-308.
[http://dx.doi.org/10.1080/10408398.2011.633249] [PMID: 24564587]

[85] Newman DJ, Cragg GM. Natural products as sources of new drugs from 1981 to 2014. J Nat Prod 2016; 79(3): 629-61.
[http://dx.doi.org/10.1021/acs.jnatprod.5b01055] [PMID: 26852623]

[86] Islam MT, Sarkar C, El-Kersh DM, *et al.* Natural products and their derivatives against coronavirus: A review of the non-clinical and pre-clinical data. Phytother Res 2020; 34(10): 2471-92.
[http://dx.doi.org/10.1002/ptr.6700] [PMID: 32248575]

[87] Ravishankar B, Shukla VJ. Indian systems of medicine: a brief profile. Afr J Tradit Complement Altern Med 2008; 4(3): 319-37.
[http://dx.doi.org/10.4314/ajtcam.v4i3.31226] [PMID: 20161896]

[88] Dev S. Ethnotherapeutic and modern drug development: The potential of Ayurveda. Curr Sci 1997; 73(11): 909-28.

[89] Mogensen TH. Pathogen recognition and inflammatory signaling in innate immune defenses. Clin Microbiol Rev 2009; 22(2): 240-73.
[http://dx.doi.org/10.1128/CMR.00046-08] [PMID: 19366914]

CHAPTER 3

Impact Of The COVID-19 Pandemic: A Changed World

Umang Tandon[1,*] and **Apoorva Tandon**[2]

[1] *Department of Commerce, Isabella Thoburn College, Lucknow, India*

[2] *Department of Computer Science, Krishna Institute of Engineering and Technology, Group of Institutions, Ghaziabad, India*

Abstract: Coronavirus disease-2019 (COVID-19) is predicted to have long-term consequences on the world's physical, mental and economic levels. June 2020 Global Economic Prospects describe the immediate and near-term impact of the pandemic, additionally the long-term injury to growth prospects. The baseline forecast predicts a 5.2% contraction in world GDP, despite the efforts made by governments to combat the downswing aided by business and financial support. Half the world's 3.3 billion personnel are threatened by the loss of their jobs. Moreover, workers within the informal economy are significantly vulnerable as a result of the lack of social protection, access to quality health care and productive assets. Individuals are finding it troublesome to survive through imprisonment as a result of a lack of resources to earn a living. According to Moody, the economic impact of the recent increase in COVID-19 cases is going to be restricted from April to June quarter, with a robust rebound within the last half of the year. The slower growth rate, on the other hand, can impede near-term economic recovery and have an impression on long-term growth dynamics. This study is focused on determining the critical effects of a Coronavirus pandemic on the global economy and anticipating the scenario that would confront the global economy soon. This research examines the various elements of Coronavirus and its economic implications.

Keywords: COVID-19, GDP, Global Economy, Global Supply Chain, Growth, Market Charge, Pandemic, Productivity, Recovery.

INTRODUCTION

The 1918 Spanish influenza, HIV/AIDS outbreaks, SARS (Severe Acute Metabolic Process Syndrome), MERS (Middle East Metabolic Process Syndrome) and Ebola are all epidemics that have unfolded throughout human history. COVID-19 was designated a global health emergency by the World Health

* **Corresponding author Umang Tandon:** Department of Commerce, Isabella Thoburn College, Lucknow, India; E-mail: umangtandon2311@gmail.com

Tahmeena Khan & Alfred J. Lawrence (Eds.)

Organization in January 2020 and a pandemic on March 11, the highest grade of medical crisis [1]. Since then, the situation has escalated into a worldwide public health and economic calamity, with far-reaching consequences for the world's $90 trillion economies not seen in almost a century. In a take on the John Donne poem, "No Man is an Island," the viral illness spread through and across countries and touched nearly every community, highlighting the global economy's interconnected nature. In March 2020, the epicentre of transmissions had moved from China to Europe, mainly Italy, but by April, the focus switched to the United States, where infection rates escalated manifold. By April 2021, viral hotspots had arisen in India, Brazil, and parts of Africa and Asia, with infection and fatality rates reaching new highs [2].

In the shortterm, every country's healthcare system has a limited capacity of ICUs, hospital beds, number of medics and paramedics, ventilators, *etc*. This puts a limit on the number of patients who can be treated successfully. Flattening the infection curve, that is, reducing the incidence of contamination and infections, is crucial to preventing clinical hospital capacity overflow in third-world countries, as well as the mortality toll that entails. When a considerable proportion of the population lives in slums, social distancing regulations become more difficult to apply, making it more difficult to control the spread. While high-income nations have an average of more than four hospital beds per thousand inhabitants, low-income countries have as few as 0.5, making it all the more difficult to treat critically ill patients [3]. This factor made coronavirus a major threat to developing countries.

THE CORONAVIRUS CURVES

The pandemic curve (Fig. **1**) also promotes a recession curve (Fig. **2**), which must also be addressed. The impacts of the disease are disruptive, and they may leave scars that prevent the economy from returning to its pre-shock state. While doing nothing damages demand and supply, social-distancing policies have exacerbated the problem [3]. Even though some people can work from home, they only make up a small percentage of the entire workforce. The masses whose income is dependent on their physical mobility are disproportionately affected by lockdowns and social isolation regulations. Another problem arises from the informality of labour in emerging countries, where the shadow economy accounts for 50% to 90% of total employment. Welfare benefits, health insurance, and paid holidays are not available to informal workers. Due to this informality of work, policies aiming at formal work, such as expanding unemployment insurance, lowering payroll taxes, and extending paid medical leave, leave a limited impact on the overall economy [3].

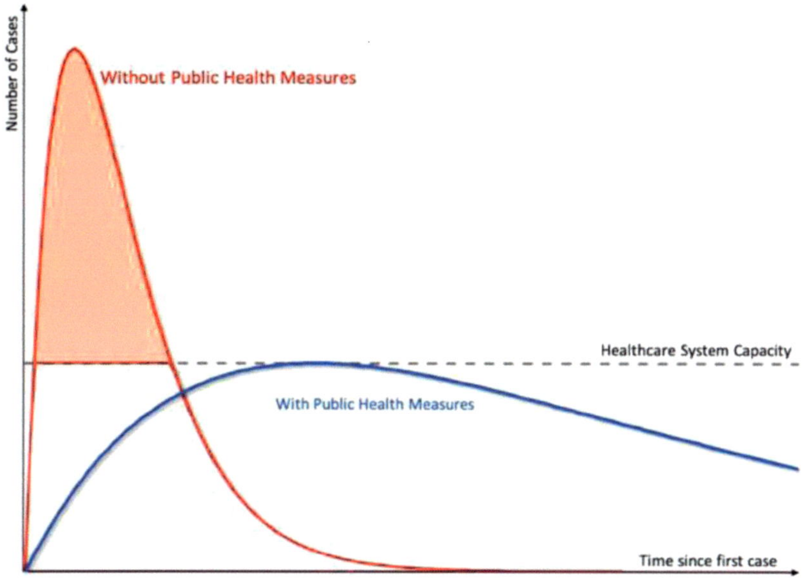

Fig. (1). The Pandemic Curve [**Source:** Gourinchas (2020)].

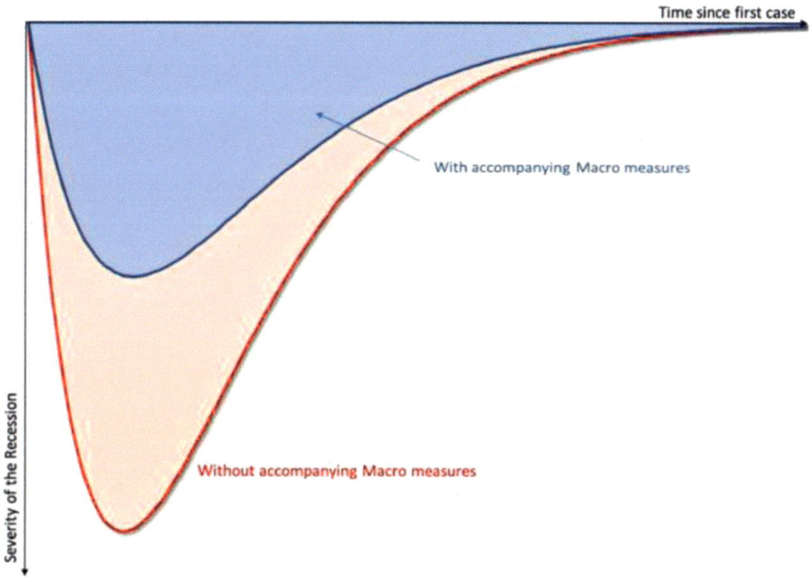

Fig. (2). The Recession Curve [**Source:** Gourinchas (2020)].

ECONOMIC IMPACT

Since the outbreak, the effects of the disease have been felt beyond mortality and morbidity in the present-day strongly connected world [4]. This has already been labelled a "Black Swan" catastrophe for the world economy by experts. Global supply networks have been hampered as the economy slows and output is disrupted. The fact that international transportation is restricted, if not prohibited, has slowed global economic activity even further. Industries relying on imports have seen massive output disruptions. Most notably, consumer and industry panic has disrupted regular shopping habits and created market anomalies. Global financial markets have also responded, with global stock indices collapsing as a result of the events [4] (Fig. **3**). Within months, tens of millions of people were laid off, and millions of small firms, as well as their suppliers, went out of business. The retail footstep (Fig. **4**) has suffered unprecedented falls as buyers continue to restrict regular outings. The situation has been amplified by new mutations and an increase in cases.

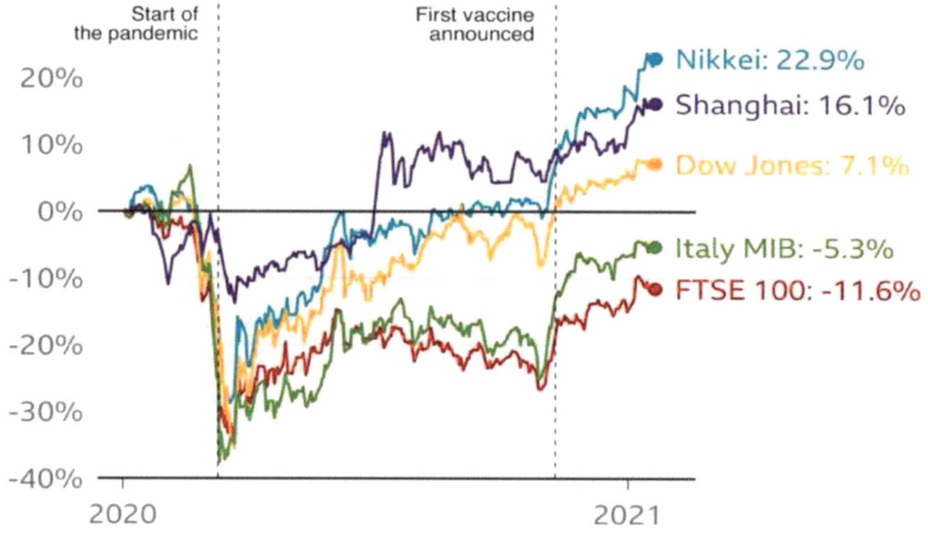

Fig. (3). Impact on Stock Markets [**Source:** Bloomberg (2021)].

What is to be seen is how severe will the decline be, and when will the economy start to recover. The recession could be a double-dip, also known as a W-shaped downturn, in which the economy falls twice before recovering to its previous growth rate, or an L-shaped situation, also known as a 'depression,' in which the economy falls steeply and does not recover for several years. So far, all studies state that the crisis will most likely mirror the L-shaped situation. We shouldn't expect things to get back to normal very soon [5].

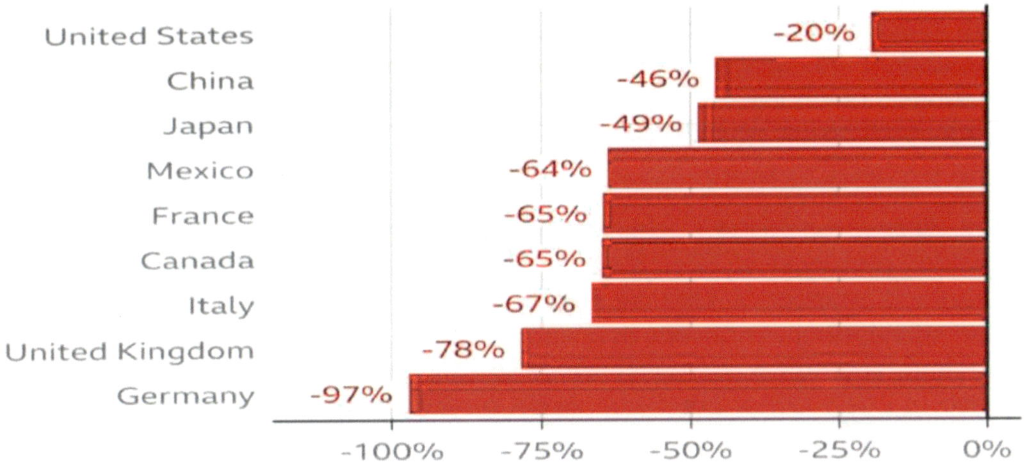

Fig. (4). Percentage change in retail footfall, 12-28 Jan 2021 *vs*. same dates in 2020 [**Source:** ShopperTrak (2021)].

"This is no longer only a global health crisis; it is also a major labour market and economic crisis that is having a huge impact on people."

Guy Ryder, Director of the International Labour Organisation

Effect on the Global Supply Chain

Global manufacturing supply chains have become more diverse and interlinked over the last few decades as globalization has accelerated and global trade volumes have increased. The Western world has grown accustomed to sourcing raw materials and finished goods from emerging economies, where cheap labour and low freight costs have made offshore supply chains viable in an age of rising expenses. Manufacturers in a variety of industries have reduced physical stocks, relying on rapid and convenient delivery of parts and a supply chain ecosystem that operates seamlessly from raw material to finished output. The combination of more efficient manufacturing methods and cheaper production costs was too enticing for many manufacturers to pass up. The advent of COVID-19, as well as the resulting global disruptions and shifts in consumption patterns, has posed a substantial challenge to supply chains, one that appears to be shaping a change in their future structure. Activity limits and shifting demand patterns create a perfect storm for processes that rely on continuous worldwide activity and bottlenecks [6].

COVID-19 has three basic effects: it has a direct impact on production (supply), breaks the production system and trades (supply), and has a financial effect on markets (demand) [7]. As a result, the global demand-supply network has been thrown into chaos (Fig. **5**). Some of this lost demand will be momentary, and once the pandemic has passed, customers will be able to make up for delayed expenditures, such as on travel. However, part of the demand will be lost indefinitely, slowing global economic growth in the long run.

In Asia, where there is less mechanization and more reliance on manual labour than in other areas of the world, COVID-19's impact on the workforce has been particularly problematic. Even though production centres in nations such as China were able to reopen in 2020 after the early viral outbreak, power disruptions, scarcity of shipping containers, and truck drivers caused manufacturing to drop in 2021. And, according to supply chain specialists, the situation is unlikely to improve in 2022. Other Southeast Asian manufacturing hubs, such as Vietnam, Malaysia, and Thailand, experience similar shortages. Sri Lanka, Bangladesh, Myanmar, Indonesia, Albania, and Central America are all seeing factory closures. By claiming force majeure clauses in contracts, European retailers have cancelled an estimated USD 1.5 billion worth of orders from Bangladesh, affecting over 1,000 garment factories. Workers who have already been hit by late paychecks and who are indebted to recruiters, risk being laid off and losing all of their immediate and long-term earnings. Businesses have pushed salary cutbacks and dismissed vulnerable workers who have little recourse against their employers [8].

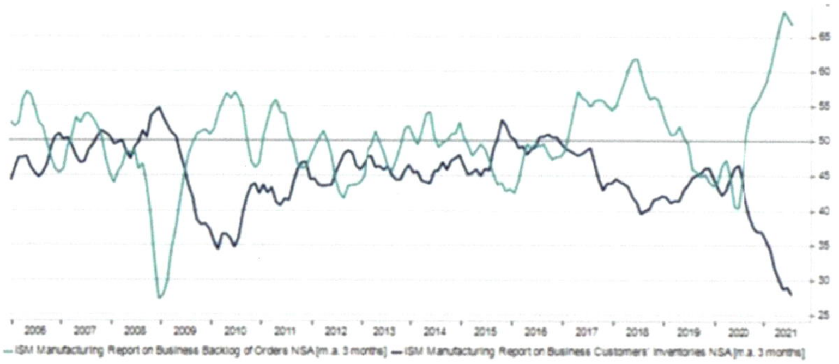

Fig. (5). ISM: The business backlog of orders, Customer Inventories [**Source:** Macrobond].

Effect on Employment and Workforce Disparities

The initial wave of job losses during the pandemic was significant, with over 20 million jobs lost between March and April 2020 (Figs. **6** - **8**). This is far greater than any prior post-war recession's losses over comparable periods. The April unemployment rate has skyrocketed since the 1930s Great Depression. According to the ILO's current predictions, there will be 52 million fewer jobs globally in 2022 than there were in the final quarter of 2019, just before the pandemic struck.

This is up from 26 million in the organization's last labour market analysis in May 2021 [9].

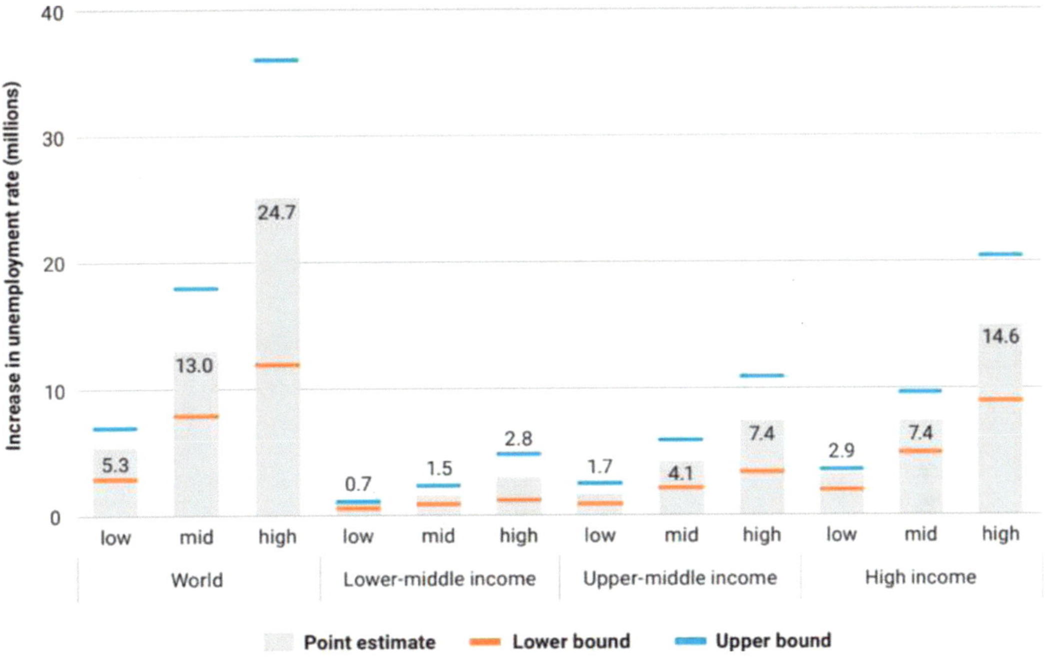

Fig. (6). Impact of Declining Global Growth on Unemployment Based on Three Scenarios, World and Income Groups (Millions) [**Source:** ILO].

"The world economy is simultaneously facing COVID-19, inflation, and policy uncertainty, with government spending and monetary policies in uncharted territory. Rising inequality and security challenges are particularly harmful to developing countries."

David Malpass, President of the World Bank Group.

Women have been disproportionately impacted by the recession, with an estimated 5% drop in female employment compared to 3.9 percent for men. According to the ILO, a greater percentage of women stepped out of the labour force, becoming inactive, as a consequence of "additional household obligations" imposed by lockdowns, which resulted in the are-rationalization of gender roles. Youth employment has also suffered as a result of the economic downturn, falling 8.7 percent in 2020 *versus* 3.7 percent for adults. This is partly because a majority of these youth worked in sectors that have been hit the hardest by social-distance limitations and lockdowns, such as retail, hospitality and recreation. Minimal-wage employees and those of black, Asian, and minority ethnic (BAME) origins have been hit especially hard, increasing concerns that the crisis's long-term impact would be to worsen inequalities [10].

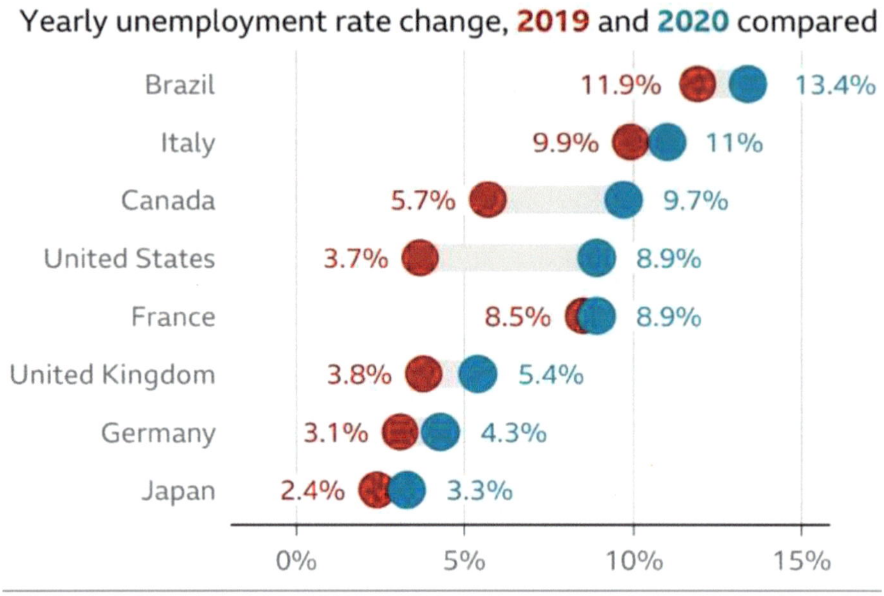

Fig. (7). Yearly unemployment rate change, 2019 *vs*. 2020 [**Source:** International Monetary Fund].

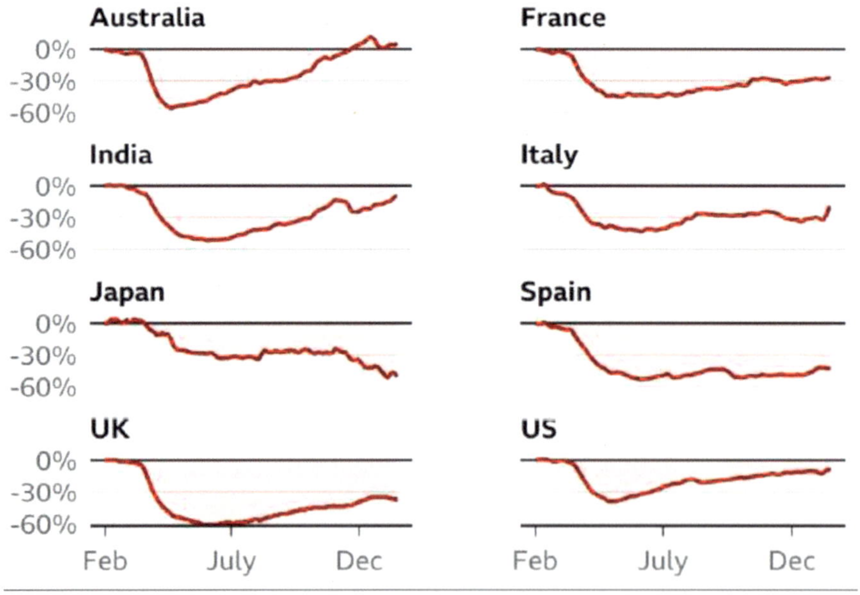

Fig. (8). Percentage change in the number of job postings, 2019 *vs*. 2020 [**Source:** Indeed.com (2021)].

According to a recent World Bank report, the developed economies' output will have largely healed by 2023, while production in emerging and developing economies will remain 4% below pre-pandemic levels. In unstable and conflict-affected countries, the impact will be substantially severe, with output slipping 7.5 percent below pre-pandemic levels. While the economic rebound in 2021 was impressive, it is expected to drop sharply from 5.5 percent last year to 4.1 percent in 2022 and 3.2 percent in 2023. In the medium term, the COVID-19 pandemic will continue to hamper economic activity, according to the Global Economic Prospects report, due to the fast spread of the Omicron strain. According to the Global Economic Prospects report, given the rapid spread of the Omicron variant, the COVID-19 pandemic will continue to disrupt economic activity in the short term [11].

GDP growth (Fig. **9**) has been the poorest since the 1950s. At the same time, debt levels have skyrocketed, particularly in developing countries. According to the IMF, the aggregate debts of the 30 largest developing economies have reached US$ 72.5 trillion, a 168 percent growth in the last ten years [5].

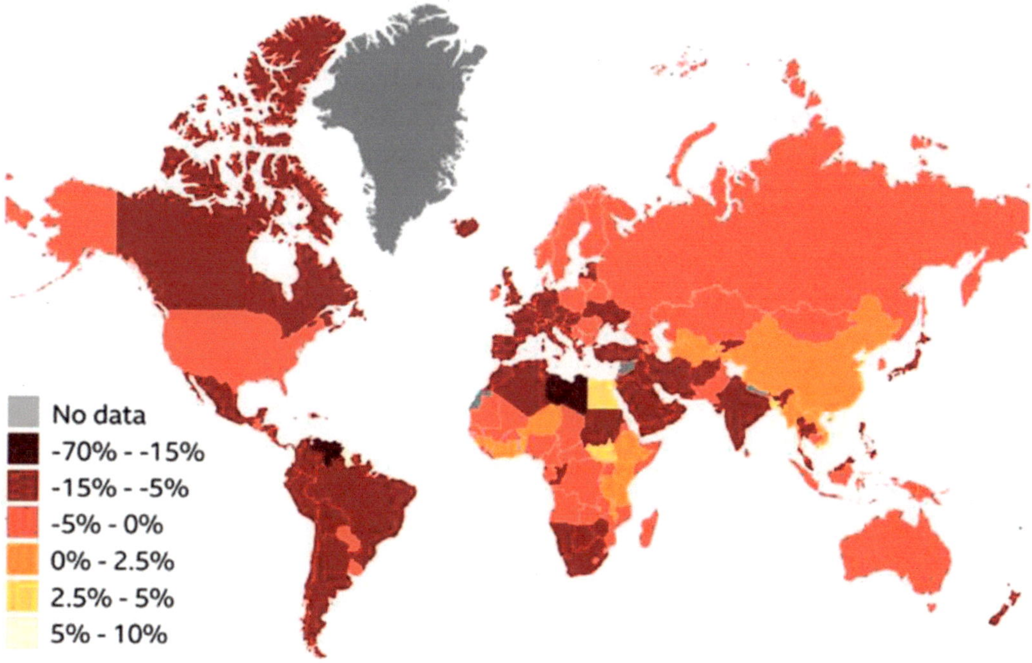

Fig. (9). GDP Growth, 2020 [**Source:** International Monetary Fund].

The crisis has reversed years of labour-market progress and, if left ignored, would increase disparities in decent work, particularly for vulnerable employees and enterprises. The most severe drop has been in middle-income countries, where the implications of this delay and disruption "may last for years," per the ILO.

Effect on Tourism and Hospitality

Tourism is amongst the most significant income drivers, especially in emerging economies, since it creates jobs, promotes inclusion and enriches cultures. It also aids the government in terms of income tax collection and foreign currency gains [12]. The COVID-19 pandemic has had a significant impact on the tourism sector (Fig. **10**). This crisis is likely to last in the medium and long term, thus countries where tourism is a major source of income, will take longer to recover. Countries that rely heavily on tourism have low levels of trade, and have a high rate of the virus are particularly vulnerable to this impact. Tourism-dependent Small Islands and Developing States (SIDS) are the worst hit by the crisis, with nations including the Maldives, Turks and Caicos, St. Lucia, Fiji, Barbados, Dominica, The Bahamas, Antigua & Barbuda, Mauritius, Cabo Verde, Belize, Grenada, St. Kitts & Nevis, and Seychelles all reporting a significant decline in GDP, ranging from 11 percent (Seychelles) to 32 percent (Maldives) (World Bank, 2021) (Fig. **11**). The pandemic is expected to inflict a 50% reduction in the hotel, restaurant, and airline business, as well as an $84 billion loss in the global airline industry [13]. Deb and Nefi cited the situation in Poland, where airport traffic was reduced by 80% and hotel occupancy rates were reduced by 40% [14]. According to the GTBA, the pandemic will cost the business travel industry $820 billion in revenue [15].

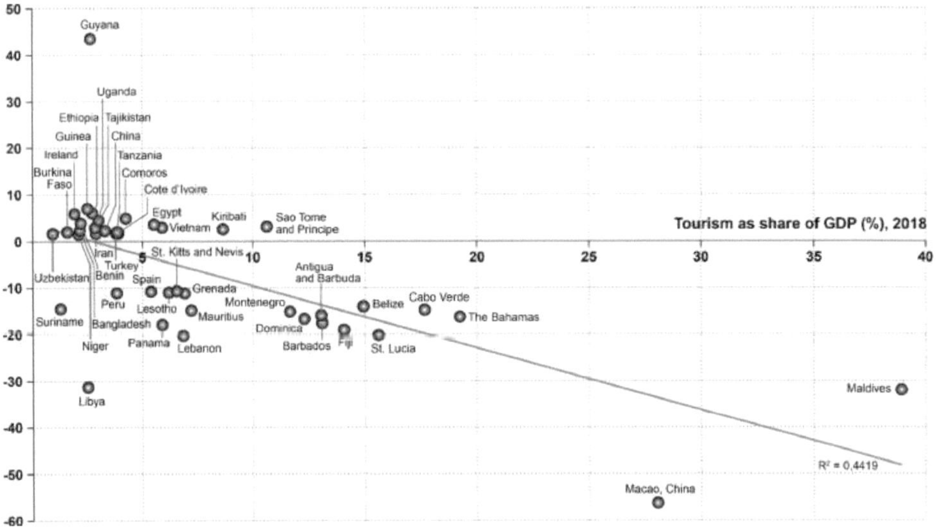

Fig. (10). Tourism Dependence and Growth/Decline in 2020 [**Source:** World Bank].

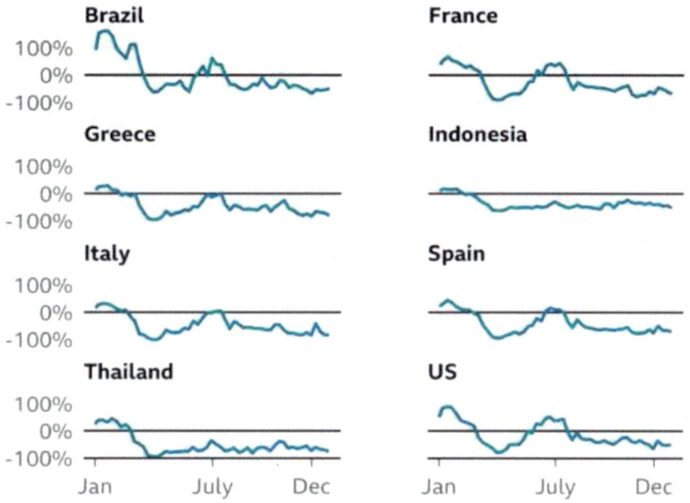

Fig. (11). Percentage change in the number of travel reservations, 2019 *vs*. 2020 [**Source:** SeeTransparent (2020)].

Along with the tourism industry's massive downturn, the food and lodging business has been among the hardest hit by the pandemic. Trade and travel restrictions have had a substantial influence on the hospitality sector's turnover. The hospitality industry's economic output in April 2020 was down 90% from February 2020. Even though output has increased after travel restrictions have been eased, it is still much below pre-pandemic levels [16]. The overall performance of this sector has been severely impacted by new strains and uncertain outbreaks.

Effect on the IT Industry

In contrast to practically all others, the IT industry has seen massive market growth, increasing from US$ 131 billion in 2020 to an estimated US$ 295 billion in the next five years. Information technology is key to delivering consistent, accurate, and dependable communication [17]. IT provides medical and economic benefits of the right to information access; additionally, IT appears to be the only way out during lockdowns and social isolation, compensating for economic and business losses. Its economic benefits in this situation have been numerous, including quick communication and innovative compensating strategies. AI-assisted virtual assistants, chatbots, and resource centres have supported the health sector in diagnosing and testing for COVID-19. Digitization has also been a key contributor to facilitating the spread of awareness and news. According to McKinsey & Company statistics, there has been a substantial change in technology adoption and digitization worldwide. As a result of the COVID-19 –

digital adoption has advanced by roughly 3 years. Since the outbreak, an estimated 35-38 percent of tech companies have strengthened or expanded their IT operations and infrastructure. The leading corporations in nearly all sectors have reported an average of a 5 to 10% rise in their IT spending. When everyone started working from home in 2020, Cloud Software and Digital Platforms had the fastest business growth. Zoom alone experienced year-on-year growth of around 340-345% in the year 2020 [18]. All of these Figs. show that the IT industry has thrived despite the global crisis, and only prevented a catastrophic shutdown in the economy.

CONCLUSION

No one can deny that COVID-19 is amongst the most serious threats the world has ever faced, with over 3.55 million individuals infected, and over a quarter of a million deaths. Billions have been put under a lockdown or have resorted to self-isolation. Despite the confusion and panic, there are growing expressions of hope and solidarity. We expect financial markets to remain erratic as the virus continues to disrupt economic activity and harm industrial and service industries worldwide. It is still unclear if this crisis will have long-term structural repercussions for the global economy or will have only short-term financial and economic consequences. The supply-demand system is in shambles. Impacts have been felt in nearly every industry, from retail to tourism and all those in between. Global economic growth has stalled, and GDP has fallen. Businesses have been shut down, jobs have been lost, and pay cuts have become common. COVID-19 is a watershed event in modern history with the ability to become a long-term impediment to economic development. The crisis is a test of the resilience of our economic, social, and medical systems, as well as the capacity of policymakers and government officials to design and implement effective strategies, the failure of which poses a formally proclaimed threat to the global economy. As outbreaks of infections are not likely to disappear anytime soon, proactive international actions are required not only to save lives but also to protect economic prosperity.

CONSENT FOR PUBLICATION

Not applicable.

CONFLICT OF INTEREST

The authors declare no conflict of interest, financial or otherwise.

ACKNOWLEDGEMENT

Declared none.

REFERENCES

[1] Chappell B. COVID-19: COVID-19 Is Now Officially a Pandemic, WHO Says 2020.https://www.npr.org/sections/goatsandsoda/2020/03/11/814474930/COVID-19-COVID-19-is-now-officiallya-pandemic-who-says

[2] Weiss M, Schwarzenberg A, Nelson R, Sutter KM, Sutherland MD. Global economic effects of COVID-19. Congressional Research Service 2020.

[3] Canuto O. The Impact of Coronavirus on The Global Economy 2020. https://media.africaportal.org/documents/Impact_of_the_coronavirus_on_global_economy.pdf

[4] McKibbin W, Fernando R. The economic impact of COVID-19. Economics in the Time of COVID-19 2020; 45: 10.1162.

[5] KALIM. "The Impact of COVID-19 on the Global economy". WORLD 2020.

[6] Supply and demand: the Covid effect 2021. https://www.nutmeg.com/nutmegonomics/supply-and-demand-the-covid-effect/

[7] Maital S, Barzani E. The global economic impact of COVID-19: A summary of research. Samuel Neaman Institute for National Policy Research 2020; 2020: 1-12.

[8] Lewery J. COVID-19: The impact on workers in global supply chains 2020. https://www.control risks.com/cOVID-19/the-impact-on-workers-in-global-supply-chains

[9] Elliot L. Covid variants have led to worse global unemployment, says ILO 2022. https://www.the guardian.com/society/2022/jan/17/covid-variants-leading-to-worse-global-unemployment-says-ilo

[10] 2021.https://news.un.org/en/story/2021/06/1093182

[11] The World Bank Group. Global Economic Prospects 2022. https://www.worldbank.org/en/publication/global-economic-prospects

[12] Jaipuria S, Parida R, Ray P. The impact of COVID-19 on tourism sector in India. Tour Recreat Res 2021; 46(2): 245-60. [http://dx.doi.org/10.1080/02508281.2020.1846971]

[13] Shaikh S, Sultan MF, Mushtaque TM, Tunio MN. Impact of COVID-19 on GDP: A Serial Mediation Effect on International Tourism and Hospitality Industry. Int J Manag 2021; 12(4): 422-30.http://www.iaeme.com/IJM/issues.asp?JType=IJM&VType=12&IType=4 [IJM].

[14] Deb, PhD Santus Kumar, and Shohel Md Nafi. Impact of COVID-19 Pandemic on Tourism: Recovery Proposal for Future Tourism (preprint). (2020).

[15] https://www.nytimes.com/reuters/2020/03/11/business/11reuters-health-coronavirus-busin-ss-travel.html

[16] Hutton G, Foley N. Hospitality industry and Covid-19, March, 2021 https://commonslibrary.parliament.uk/research-briefings/cbp-9111/

[17] Impacts of COVID-19 on the Information Technology (IT) industry, April, 2020 https://www.marketdataforecast.com/blog/impacts-of-covid19-on-information-technology-industry

[18] Impacts of Covid-19 on Information Technology (IT) Industry, June, 2021 https://www.geeksforgeeks.org/impacts-of-cOVID-19-on-information-technology-it-industry/

CHAPTER 4

Impact of COVID-19 Pandemic on Women

Tahmeena Khan[1], **Saima Arif**[2,3] and **Alfred J. Lawrence**[2,*]

[1] *Department of Chemistry, Integral University, Lucknow, 226026, U.P., India*

[2] *Department of Chemistry, Isabella Thoburn College, Lucknow, 226007, Uttar Pradesh, India*

[3] *Toxicokinetics Laboratory, CSIR- Indian Institute of Toxicology Research (IITR), Lucknow, 226001, Uttar Pradesh, India*

Abstract: SARS-CoV-2 virus, leading to the COVID-19 pandemic, was first recognized in 2019. The impact of the crisis is never gender-neutral, and COVID-19 is no exception. While everyone is facing unprecedented challenges, women bear the brunt of the economic and social fallout of COVID-19. Hygiene and nutritional aspects are important parameters for the assessment of the overall health and well-being of a person. This chapter has shed light on the impact of the COVID-19 pandemic on women and how their sanitary/hygiene routine has been impacted in the current scenario. Through an online questionnaire survey with 510 women, the overall impact on their lives, including health and hygiene and nutritional practices, is presented as a case study. 69.4% of women reported spending some time on a physical fitness regime, and 66.2% of them believed that wearing a mask can reduce the risk of infection. 56.3% of women reported no side effects related to masks, however, 25.6% of women reported breathing issues whereas, skin rashes and itching and ear pain were some other symptoms reported. Women became more careful about their health during the pandemic, and 73.1% of them reported to have consumed additional measures to boost their immunity, and 74.4% of the women reported that their fruit intake increased during the pandemic. 52.2% of the respondents also reported consuming some health supplements. The awareness can be linked to educational status as the majority of respondents had university degrees, out of which 33.5% were graduates, and 30% were post-graduates.

Keywords: COVID-19, Education, Health, Helsinki Declaration, Hygiene, Immunity, Nutrition, Physical fitness, Protection, Survey, Women.

INTRODUCTION

The novel coronavirus (COVID-19) or SARS-CoV-2 pandemic started in Wuhan, China, at the end of 2019 and spread over the world by 2020. In the absence of

* **Corresponding author Alfred J. Lawrence:** Department of chemistry, Isabella Thoburn College, Lucknow-226007, Uttar Pradesh, India: E-mail: Alfred_lawrence@yahoo.com

any concrete medicinal solutions, various preventive measures like social distancing and massive lockdowns have been implemented by governments, resulting in people staying at home. The lockdowns also saw closures of educational institutions, offices, gyms and other non-essential services [1]. The pandemic has not only posed a threat to human health, but it has also had an impact on human existence at all levels, resulting in economic losses and jeopardising mental health. The current situation's societal impacts are partly discriminatory and gender prejudiced, notably affecting the marginalised population and women. The "care economy" has been severely disrupted, rendering women more vulnerable to bear the effects of the situation not just now, but also in the near future [2]. Gender is a social predictor of health [3], and women report more unhealthy days on average, both emotionally and physically, than males [4]. Asthma, diabetes, and myocardial infarction are examples of health issues.

Health conditions like asthma, diabetes and myocardial infarctions [5] are often encountered by women, particularly those belonging to less privileged socioeconomic classes, and those belonging to the rural background and low educational profiles [6]. The coronavirus pandemic is expected to plunge 47 million women into poverty, according to United Nations research. According to the report, while the pandemic will have a worldwide impact on poverty, it will disproportionately affect women. By 2021, there will be 118 women for every 100 men aged 25 to 34 living in extreme poverty (on less than $1.90 per day), with the difference anticipated to widen to 121 women for every 100 men by 2030 [https://www.unwomen.org//media/headquarters/attachments/sections/library/publications/2020/gender-equality-in-the-wake-of-covid-19-en.pdf?l a=en&vs =5142].

COVID-19 and its Impact

Severe acute respiratory syndrome coronavirus 2 (SARS-CoV-2) is the root cause of the ongoing COVID -19 pandemic. In 2019, the SARS-CoV-2 virus, which is closely related to the SARS-CoV virus, caused an outbreak of Novel coronavirus disease. Since its first instance was discovered in December 2019 in Wuhan, China, COVID-19 has rapidly spread over the world, claiming 1,692,230 deaths as of December 20, 2020 [7]. Between 31st December 2019 to 20th December 2020, 76,738,133 cases have been reported so far. The history of coronavirus dates back to 1965 when it was first identified by scientists in humans which led to the common cold. The term "Coronavirus" has been derived from the Latin word Corona which translates to "crown" in English owing to its structural morphology. A novel severe acute respiratory syndrome (SARS) was reported from Southern China in 2002 and 2003, and it spread to around 29 nations. A total of 8098 people were affected, with 774 deaths reported [8]. The COVID-19 pandemic has wreaked havoc on the population, causing acute health concerns mostly related to respiratory disorders, which include symptoms such as dry cough, fever, sore throat, and loss of taste and smell. Since the outset of the COVID-19 pandemic, the number of new confirmed cases and deaths has been growing continuously, with a global fatality rate of 2.20% and a recovery rate of 70.19% [7]. The current global statistics of the COVID-19 as of 23rd January 2022 are represented in Table **1**. India stands second in the list of the most number of confirmed cases with a mortality rate of 1.45%. The worst-hit Indian states have been summarized in Table **2**.

Table 1. COVID-effect in ten worst-hit countries as of 23rd January 2022 (https://www.worldometers.info/coronavirus /countries-where-coronavirus-has-spread/).

Country	Population	Total Tests	Total Cases	Total Recovered	Total Deaths
USA	334024770	879598015	71,728,557	43892277	489,422
India	1401124519	715520580	39,237,264	35807029	622,979
Brazil	214911839	63776166	23,960,207	21848301	128,514
France	65498431	222105082	16,390,818	9612731	153,787
UK	68441263	440125448	15,784,488	11738323	326,112
Russia	146031913	247600000	11,108,191	9925855	85,784
Turkey	85751692	127511700	10,881,626	9899648	143,296
Italy	60323364	162273201	9,781,191	6450596	91,741
Spain	46782980	66213858	8,975,458	5390818	117,323
Germany	84201113	89622218	8,641,865	7139800	119,103

Table 2. Details of Worst COVID-19 Hit Ten States in India (https://www.covid19india.org/).

State	Population (In crore)	Total Testings (In crore)	Total Cases	Total Recovered	Total Deaths
Maharashtra	12.2	6.3	6611078	6450585	140216
Kerala	3.5	3.8	4968657	4857181	31681
Karnataka	6.6	5.1	2988333	2941578	38082
Tamil Nadu	7.6	5.1	2702623	2655015	36116
Andhra Pradesh	5.2	3	2066450	2047722	14373
Uttar Pradesh	22.5	8.4	1710158	1687151	22900
West Bengal	9.7	1.9	1592908	1565471	19141
Delhi	2	2.9	1439870	1414431	25091
Odisha	4.4	2.2	1041457	1029147	8386

(Table 2) cont.....

State	Population (In crore)	Total Testings (In crore)	Total Cases	Total Recovered	Total Deaths
Chhattisgarh	2.9	1.4	1006052	992159	13577

Effect of COVID -19 Pandemic on the Human Race

To curb the spread of coronavirus, measures like physical distancing, regular washing of hands and usage of face masks, *etc*., were suggested. A handful of countries imposed nationwide lockdowns, of which China was the very first nation to do so. About half of the world was under lockdown around April 2020. On one hand where the well-to-do citizens, stable in terms of finances, jobs, residents and nutrition, isolated themselves in their homes; racial minorities, migrant labourers, daily wagers, and people from weaker financial backgrounds were in grave mental trauma; on the other hand, owing to the loss of financial means and security [9]. The virus has been addressed as a “great equalizer” in view that it affects anyone irrespective of the person’s caste, creed, race, gender or social status and is not discriminating. However, a difference in opinion arises due to an enormous variance in access to resources necessary for survival amongst discrete social groups. From 25th March 2020, the first phase of a complete nationwide lockdown started in India. Having lost their jobs, hundreds of thousands of hungry and helpless migrant labourers continued to march towards their native places. According to the International Labour Organization (ILO), around 400 million jobs were lost worldwide between April 2020 and June 2020 due to the COVID-19 pandemic [10]. Moreover, the people who worked as “essential workers” faced problems about the lack of proper health measures, safety equipment, extremely long working hours, emotional exhaustion and excessive workload, *etc*. People's psychological well-being has also suffered as a result of the COVID-19 epidemic. Fear of contracting the virus, being separated from family, stress, anxiety, hopelessness during the lockdown, financial instability, uncertainty about the pandemic situation's outcome, boredom, loneliness, and the development of suicidal tendencies are just a few of the psychological traits that people experienced during the pandemic [11]. The people who contracted the virus suffered from stigmatization and faced rejection from society, once they recovered.

Women and COVID 19

While women were already handling the majority of the world's unpaid care work before the COVID-19 pandemic, a new study reveals that the crisis and its following shutdown reaction resulted in a significant rise in this burden. Without early action, the detrimental effects on women and families are likely to linger for years [12]. According to a report released by United Nations, the burden of unpaid work has increased substantially, which is of particular importance to the women who are engaged in meeting the needs of the family, caring for the older members of the household and taking care of household chores [13]. Although the lockdown period has been fruitful in some instances, like in Japan, the suicide rate has lowered as compared to 2019, as people spent more time with family [14]. According to another survey-based study in the United Kingdom, 80% of the respondents formed a stronger bond with family members owing to the closeness experienced during the lockdown [15]. In addition to these positive outcomes, the responses also hint towards inequalities and gender biases faced during this tough time. The burden of unpaid labour has risen for women as schools and nurseries have closed, and their participation in economic stability has become more precarious than ever. Working couples are being forced to make difficult decisions about who will care about the home and children as the burden of unpaid labour grows. This added load has hampered women's capacity to work, which is mostly owing to conventional gender roles and a regressive belief that women's economic contributions are often part-time, flexible, and low-paying [16]. The situation for women has been made more difficult by the colour and caste systems. According to a recent survey in the United States, more than a third of women have been laid off or have had salary cutbacks as a result of the coronavirus pandemic, and the situation is much more problematic for black women, who are 54% more likely than white males to lose their jobs [17]. Women are less likely to be able to afford necessities for more than a month due to job insecurity, and black women are far more likely than white men to report financial insecurity [17]. The pattern is similar to that seen in previous pandemics such as SARS, swine flu, and birds blue, all of which had long-term negative effects on women, both on and off the job. Reports from the USA suggest that parents are skeptical to take their wards for vaccinations and routine health check-ups, which may exacerbate childhood illness in the future [18], which is as likely to take a toll on their mothers' overall health and financial well-being.

Women and Health and Hygiene

The current pandemic prevented about 1·52 billion children from attending school, as estimated by UNESCO in March 2020, and some of them would never return [19]. Schools provide a secure environment for vulnerable girls by providing sanitary amenities such as towels and sanitary napkins, as well as a protected atmosphere free of abuse that they may suffer at home. The loss of this protection might have serious health consequences, including teen pregnancy and sexually transmitted diseases. Women are forced to provide unpaid labour, domestic duties, childcare, preparing food for the extra children who would normally be at school, and looking after sick family members as their access to paid work diminishes as a result of the lockdown and school closures, and these responsibilities fall disproportionately on women.

Reproductive Health

According to a maternity centre, nearly 9.5 million women are less inclined to attend the centre for safe abortions and contraception, mostly owing to their fear of contracting the virus and as a COVID-19 control measure. As a result of the impediment in visits, malnourished infants are expected to be born in the future [19]. According to the Foundation for Reproductive Health Services in India, 26 million Indian couples were unable to access contraception as a result of the lockdown, resulting in 2.3 million unwanted pregnancies and over 800,000 unsafe abortions, the third leading cause of maternal deaths in the country [20].

Psychological Health

The pandemic has also made an impact on psychological health and well-being, having a biased effect on women. Depression and anxiety are commonly associated with one in seven women during the perinatal period which is linked to reduced mother-infant bonding. This may be diagnosed and the treatment is critical, yet it is reported that 50% of the women who suffer from depression remain undiagnosed [21]. In Italy, a survey of 100 pregnant women showed a varying impact on mental health, which needs medical intercession [22]. Women Health workers from countries like Bangladesh, India and Mexico have reported violent attacks, harassment and abuse, mostly due to the result of misunderstanding and lack education and information [23]. This may affect mental health and low morale at the workplace and fear of safety concerns. Another study conducted in Hubei Province, China, showed that women suffered from more post-traumatic symptoms than men in the aftermath of the pandemic [24]. Another study conducted with US individuals showed that women experienced more stress-inducing events than men during the COVID-19 outbreak [25]. Lockdown and physical distancing has seen a sharp rise in domestic and sexual violence, as women have been trapped with their abuser. Emerging data has shown that the complaints related to domestic violence increased during the pandemic owing to heightened stress, tension, financial insecurities, and health concerns. It has been estimated that 15 million additional cases of gender-based violence are going to occur globally till restrictions of movement are in place [26]. Intimate partner violence has also been associated with higher morbidity and mortality for co-occurring diseases [27]. A survey conducted in May 2020 highlighted the pathos of the victims and their difficulty and inaccessibility to resources and showed that the survivors are under increased strain [28]. The Young Women's Christian Association (YMCA) USA, has reported almost full shelters across the USA, at the peak of the pandemic, with a high risk of viral transmission [29]. Findings of a large-scale survey suggest that women with no social connections and in need of social support are more likely to suffer from adverse mental health consequences and outcomes [30].

Nutritional Aspects Concerning Women's Health

According to the World Food Program, the pandemic has led to a food crisis. The disruptions caused in the markets and international trade will make an impact in the long run as well, with approximately 265 million people facing the threat of hunger and malnutrition [31]. Households-led women are more at risk of starvation as women constitute a share of 60% of the food-deprived lot globally. After clubbing the rise in gender-based violence and other implications of COVID-19, the potential impacts are overwhelming [32]. On a global basis, 80-90% of women are involved in cooking. They are also involved in grocery shopping and spend most of their earnings in providing food for their families. They are also accountable for providing child care. In case of an emergent crisis, women are the first who sacrifice their share of food, to support their families. In such a situation when the hunger pandemic hits, women are more likely to have fewer nutrients which are essential for strengthening the immune system to fight against infections. Women belonging to developing countries, for example, India, do not have the proper means to satiate their food demand.

On average, at reproductive age, an Indian woman has a body mass index (BMI) that is lower than 18.5 kg/m [33]. Approximately 53% of women in India are anaemic, and 31% and 37% have vitamin B12 and folate deficiency [34]. There are many reasons responsible for the food crisis, including lack of education, access to primary health facilities and nutrition services, *etc.* The situation has only worsened during the pandemic leading to a downfall in the health of women. Table **3** represents the dietary recommended levels of some essential nutrients for women [35].

Table 3. Daily recommended levels of some nutrients for women.

S.No.	NUTRIENTS	RECOMMENDATIONS	
		HEALTHY WOMAN	DISEASED WOMAN
1	Vitamin C	200 mg/day	1-2 g/day
2	Vitamin D	200 IU/day	10,000 IU/week
3	Vitamin E	15 mg/day	200 IU/day
4	Selenium	50 μg/day	Upto 200 μg/day
5	Zinc	11 mg/day	75 mg/day

(Table 3) cont.....

S.No.	NUTRIENTS	RECOMMENDATIONS	
		HEALTHY WOMAN	DISEASED WOMAN
6	Iron	Women age 19-50: 18mg/day Women age>51: 8 mg/day	60 mg Fe/day
7	Omega-3 Fatty Acids(Epa+Dha)	250-300 mg/day of EPA+DHA	1500-3000 mg/day of EPA+ DHA
8	Multivitamin Supplements including Vitamins (A,B6,B12,C,D,E & Folate) & Trace Elements (Zn, Fe, Mg & Cu)	Supplying nutrient requirements according to the 100% RDA for age & gender. This is in addition to a well balanced diet.	

The Impact of the Pandemic on Indian Women

The occurrence of COVID-19 in India has bought unprecedented losses. Women and girls, and marginalized groups are at a greater risk without having any means to absorb the economic shocks and mitigation strategies to address the health crisis as they are the primary caregivers and also extending efforts to sustain livelihood amidst the lurking threat of a third wave. Although, women constitute a noteworthy percentage of all healthcare workers, however in decision-making, they are not accounted for. According to a study conducted by Dalberg Advisors, it was found that the pandemic 28% of Indian women accounted for job losses during the pandemic, even though 24% of them contributed to the workforce. They devote ten times more time to household chores as compared to their male counterparts. Owing to this disparity, two-thirds of their income was lost and the household burden amplified during the pandemic, making it more difficult to take up employment again, which will have poor economic outcomes. The study also reported that health and nutritional conditions are often unreported, which affect every single woman out of four belonging to the low-income group [https://dalberg.com/our-ideas/the-disproportionate-impact-of-covid-19-on-women-in-india/]. It has also been reported that women found it difficult to access menstrual hygiene products, particularly in rural regions. Unplanned pregnancies have also been reported to surge among women belonging to low-income households, particularly due to their lack of access to precautionary measures. The issue of domestic violence also came into the spotlight as the National Commission for Women (NCW) reported a 100% rise in complaints of violence against women within a fortnight of the first phase of the lockdown in India [https://en.unesco.org/ news/women-centre-unescos-covid-19-response-india]. A hike in domestic violence was reported during March and April 2020 as reported by the NCW as compared to February [https://www.google.com/ search ?q=domestic+violence+in+india+during+lockdown&oq=Domestic+violence+in+ &aqs=chrome.4.69i57j0l7.12809j0j8&sourceid=chrome&ie= UTF-8]. In Punjab an approximate 21% rise in domestic violence, cases was reported. States like Uttar Pradesh, Bihar and Haryana also reported a surge in such complaints. [https://www.theweek.in/news/india/2020/04/23/700-domestic-violence-cases-registered-during-lockdown-in-punjab.html]. Along with these issues, women and girls need an iron-rich diet, and they are usually offered bland, nutrition reduced diet leading to problems like anaemia in approximately 53% of the Indian women aged between 15-49. The socio-economic impact on women will have future outcomes calling for exclusive strategies and administrative support for women. Data released by the United Nations has shown that the percentage of girls quitting school was more and 65% of the parents were hesitant to send them back to school. The lack of education, information and resources makes women more susceptible to catching the COVID-19 infection. The discrimination in the percentage of women getting vaccinated as compared to men is another challenge to overcome. According to the latest data, 17% of men are more vaccinated than women. Women may be lagging as they may not have internet accessibility and do not possess phones and hence are unable to get themselves registered for vaccination. Patriarchal norms also hold back women from going to the vaccination centres alone. The government of India, through a mobile App "Aarogya Setu" generates automatic messages and information about the viral symptoms, risk factors and promotes preventive behaviours and measures like washing hands, usage of masks, and maintaining social distance, but there is no research to trace out how this message is being received and implemented by men and women or which group is taking the measures more seriously. A study conducted in the South Asia region (excluding India) found that women are more likely to miss such information than men [36]. Access to the internet, smartphone and literacy rate is lower in women than men in India [37]. Access and understanding of health promotion messages must be supported by making resources available to access the internet [38]. These gender-based issues and gaps make women and girls more vulnerable and cause lesser adaption of healthy practices. India has the majority of adolescents and young adults the world over, and it is very imperative to know the impact of the pandemic on them, particularly in gender stratified setting with the prevalence of gender disproportion and conventional norms affecting the well-being of women it is very critical to understand the future outcome of the pandemic. However, there is little known regarding the experience of women and girls and how they adapt to the current scenario and cope with the situation. To understand the changes in the lifestyle of women and girls an online questionnaire survey was done exclusively with women coming from different age groups and educational profiles and the study is discussed in detail in the subsequent sections.

A SURVEY-BASED STUDY WITH WOMEN

A questionnaire survey is an inexpensive and reliable method to gather data from a large sample size. An online survey was done with 510 women respondents, primarily of Indian origin, between 15th November 2020-15th December 2020 to know how their lives were impacted at different levels, including their physical fitness, sanitary and hygiene practices and nutritional aspects during the pandemic. The questionnaire was developed as a Google form and was shared through various social media sites following snowball sampling. Snowball sampling facilitates a larger number of responses and in the process, the questionnaire is shared from one participant to another and so on. It is a non-probability sampling method. The questionnaire was developed according to the guidelines by the UN's women global gender data programme, Making Every Woman and Girl Count, in response to the COVID-19 pandemic (Rapid Gender Assessment Surveys on the impact of COVID-19 Guidance documents) [https://data.unwomen.org/publications/guidance-rapid-gender-assessmen--surveys-impacts-covid19] and based on the Helsinki Declaration. The information was kept strictly confidential and only used for research purposes. No written consent was sought by the participants. Since voluntary answers were sought to maintain the interest of the respondent, a limited number of questions were made compulsory.

RESULTS AND DISCUSSION

Demographic Details

47.6% (n=243) of respondents were between 20-29 year age bracket and 38.6% respondents (n=197) were between 15-19 age group. The majority of the respondents (99.6%) were Indian nationals. Out of all the respondents, 83.9% (n=428) were single, while 15.5% (n=79) were married, the majority of them *viz.* 97.6% (n=418) had urban background whereas, 12.4% (n= 59) belonged to rural background. The majority of them (63.1%) belonged to nuclear households. The educational profile showed that 33.5% of the respondents were graduates and 30% had a post-graduate degree. Demographic details are given in Table **4**. Most of the respondents had post-secondary education.

Table 4. Demographic details of Participants.

Age of Participants		
Response	**Percentage**	**Number of Respondents**
15 - 19	38.6	197
20 - 29	47.6	243

(Table 4) cont.....

Age of Participants		
Response	**Percentage**	**Number of Respondents**
30 - 39	8.2	42
40 - 49	3.3	17
50 - 59	1.4	7
60 or above	0.8	4
Religion of Participants		
Response	**Percentage**	**Number of Respondents**
Hinduism	60.19	307
Islam	34.7	177
Christianity	4.31	22
Sikkhism	0.4	2
Others	0.4	2
Country of Residence		
Response	**Percentage**	**Number of Respondents**
India	99.21	506
Kingdom of Saudi Arabia (KSA)	0.19	1
United Arab Emirates (UAE)	0.39	2
France	0.19	1
Marital Status		
Response	**Percentage**	**Number of Respondents**
Single	83.9	428
Married	15.5	79
Separated, divorced or widowed	0.6	3
Area of Residence		
Response	**Percentage**	**Number of Respondents**
Urban	87	435
Rural	13	65
Nature of Family		
Response	**Percentage**	**Number of Respondents**
Nuclear	68.43	349
Joint	34.7	177
Total Members in the Family		
Response	**Percentage**	**Number of Respondents**
1 - 5	65.1	332

(Table 4) cont.....

Age of Participants		
Response	**Percentage**	**Number of Respondents**
5 - 10	28	143
More than 10	6.9	35
Number of Children		
Response	**Percentage**	**Number of Respondents**
None	73.1	373
1	10.2	52
2	10.4	53
3	4.7	24
4	1.6	8
Highest Education Level		
Response	**Percentage**	**Number of Respondents**
No education	0	0
High school	1	5
Intermediate	35.5	181
Graduate	33.5	171
Postgraduate and above	30	153

Employment Details

Women make up 39 percent of global employment but account for 54 percent of overall job losses (https://www.mckinsey.com/featured-insights/future-of-work/covid-19-and-gender-equality-countering-the-regressive-effects). The pandemic and the preventive measures have driven a lopsided augmentation in women's unemployment (https://www.unwomen.org/en/ news/stories/2020/9/feature-covid-19-economic- impacts-on-women). Working women have found it more difficult to balance their professional commitments with personal responsibilities. The employment details showed that of the total working respondents, 60.6% respondents were employed in the private sector and 39.4% were employed in the public sector. 37.3% (n=107) of respondents reported increased professional burden. 1.4% of the employed respondents also resigned from their job during the pandemic. 32% of employed women reported salary deductions and 57.3% reported no change in salary structure.

Physical Fitness and Nutritional Aspects

Although the pandemic has imposed a lopsided burden on women in different aspects of their daily routine, as a whole, the "stay at home" time has also encouraged them to take care of their health and pursue their hobbies and fitness regimen. This may be attributed to their social status and educational profile and living style. The survey results showed that 64.9% of respondents took out time to maintain their physical fitness (Fig. **1**), although due to paucity of time, most of the surveyed women (49.7%) spent half an hour on different physical activities, still, an appreciable percentage of 40.9% women spent an hour daily on their fitness regimen. Yoga (31.9%) was the most preferred activity, whereas aerobics, dancing and walking (37.7%) were also taken up by women (Fig. **2**). Pandemic and its concerns seemed to do a good deed when it came to paying attention to nutrition. People especially women, became more aware of what they and their families eat. It has been established that the development of COVID-19 from mild to serious symptoms is very much associated with the nutritional aspect; therefore, it is of utmost importance to assess the nutritional status in the context to COVID-19, therefore a section on "Nutritional Aspects" was included in the questionnaire. 80% of women said that they had 3 meals a day like pre-pandemic and 74.4% of women consumed more fruits (Fig. **3**) and had vitamin-rich diets (69.4%) or included vitamin supplements to strengthen their immunity (52.2%). Herbal concoctions were also added to the diet as reported by 73.1% of women.

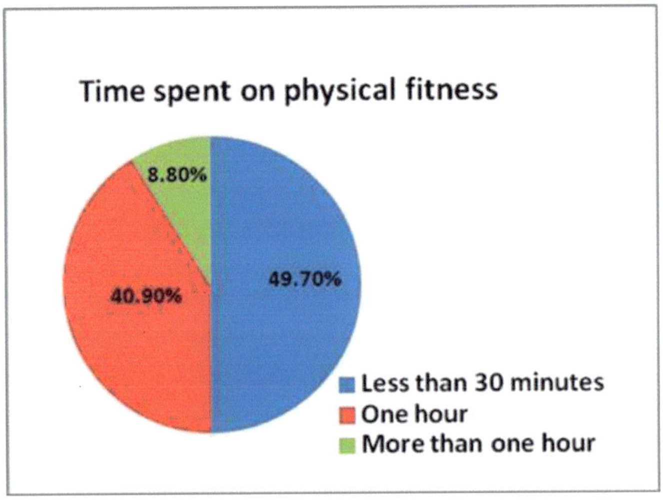

Fig. (1). Devoted time on physical activity.

Menstrual health of women is of extreme importance and the survey results portray that the pandemic phase didn't seem to have much effect on the menstruation cycle of women. 71.2% of women said to have experienced no particular change in their menstrual cycles during the lockdown period. Studies across the globe have suggested a remarkable betterment in menstrual health and the conceiving rate of women. Many studies are found to bring out the fact that a changed and balanced lifestyle during lockdown helped many women in conceiving who had been trying for quite a long time pre-pandemic. As the pandemic continues, it would be interesting to know whether physical activity or exercise might interact with the immune system to affect the infectivity and associated susceptibility of the virus. Retrospective studies are needed to see whether physical activity status has any association with the COVID-19 infection.

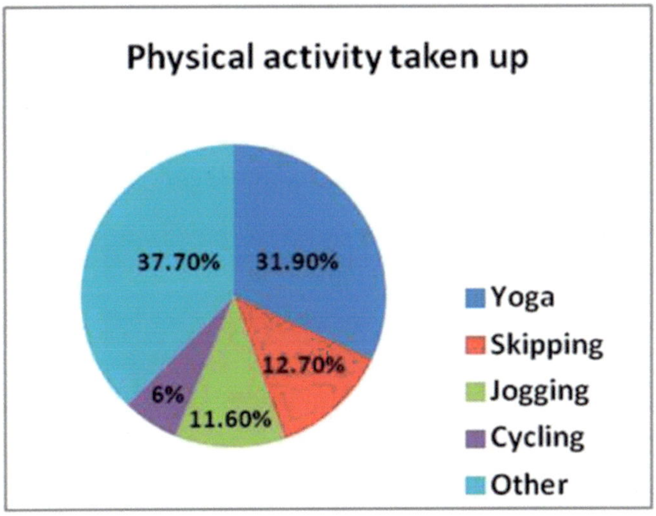

Fig. (2). Prominent reported physical activities.

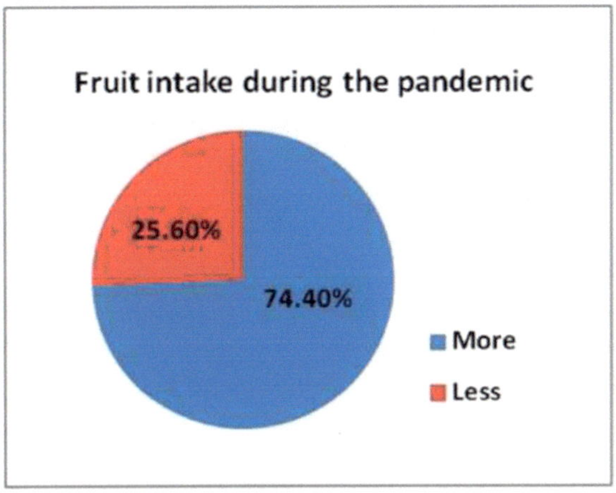

Fig. (3). Fruits consumption reported by the respondents.

Sanitary and Hygiene Practices

In the absence of concrete medicinal interventions, preventive measures like using face masks, regular washing and sanitization of hands with alcohol-based sanitisers have been encouraged. Even women have become aware of the various sanitary practices and have adapted to new sanitary practices [39] (Fig. **4**). To know how well the surveyed women adapted to the different precautionary measures, a section on sanitary practices was included. According to the findings of the survey, the majority of the women reported having spent Rs. 500-1000 every month on the procurement of face masks and sanitisers, whereas 29.1 percent (n= 116) respondents spent between Rs. 100-500 on the same. The majority of the respondents (66.2%) believed that wearing a face mask can protect them against infection. Cloth masks, used by 62% of the respondents were more common, followed by surgical masks (17.6%). They also regularly washed their cloth masks, as reported by 54.8% of respondents. Although there were no adverse consequences associated with the usage of masks, however, 25.6% of women had breathing problems, skin rashes and ear pain (Table **5**).

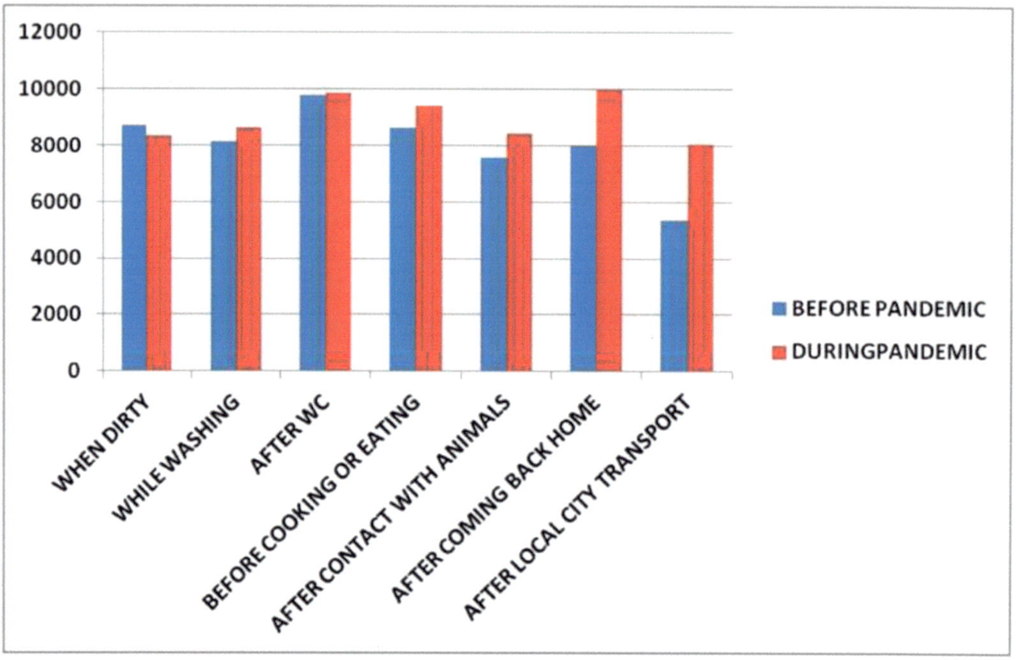

Fig. (4). Sanitary and Hygiene practices observed in Polish women during the lockdown [36].

The comprehensive online survey was conducted to assess the overall impact of the COVID-19 pandemic on women concerning changes in lifestyle, employability, health, hygiene and nutritional practices. The findings of the study revealed that women are the ones who are sharing the burden of unpaid care work at home, although the majority of the surveyed women were well-qualified. On the positive side, respondents were found to be more aware and keen to improve their health and boost their immunity. They also devoted some time daily to maintain their physical fitness and also indulged in reading or surfing social media during their free time. Similarly, they were also found to be aware and concerned for their safety as a majority of them used face masks and allocated a monthly budget for the purchase of preventive measures. The awareness may be attributed to the appreciable educational profile as the majority of the respondents had a university education and belonged to urban set-ups and belonged to nuclear households. Given the conditions of social distancing, snowball sampling was done to procure data and that may have led to the generalizability of the results. Owing to the snowball sampling, the possibility of selection bias must also be considered. Another limitation of the study was that the survey was accessed by those having internet facilities and therefore, most of the responses were received from urban dwellers. Moreover, the majority of the respondents were between 20-29 years old, and the same study must be conducted with middle-aged and elderly women who may not be internet friendly. The responses on mental health call for strengthening strategies to protect women during periods of crisis. The survey did not take into account those who chose not to participate. However, since the majority of the women belonged to urban backgrounds with sound educational backgrounds, hence they were keen to share their opinion through the provided medium. However, a lack of internet and computer knowledge may reduce the responses obtained in online surveys [40]. Another limitation of the study was that the majority of the respondents were Indian nationals, and the results could not capture a diverse population.

Table 5. Preventive measures used during the pandemic.

Prevention of COVID-19 using Face Mask (Total Responses - 491)		
Response	**Percentage**	**Number of Respondents**
Yes	66.2	325
No	2.0	10
No, but I still use to feel safe	22.4	110
Maybe	9.4	46
Comfort Level While Wearing a Mask (Total Responses - 491)		
Response	**Percentage**	**Number of Respondents**
Comfortable	44.4	218
Not so comfortable	53.4	262
Don't wear at all	1.0	5
Not so comfortable, but important	0.8	4
Very comfortable	0.4	2
Usage of the Mask Before Pandemic (Total Responses - 488)		
Response	**Percentage**	**Number of Respondents**

(Table 5) cont.....

Prevention of COVID-19 using Face Mask (Total Responses - 491)		
Response	**Percentage**	**Number of Respondents**
Yes, always	10.7	52
No, never	60.2	294
Sometimes	19.9	97
Rarely	9.2	45
Frequency of Wash and Sterilization of Mask (Total Responses - 454)		
Response	**Percentage**	**Number of Respondents**
Daily	54.8	249
Once in 3 days	19.2	87
Weekly	8.4	38
Don't wash at all	1.1	5
Don't use a cloth mask	16.5	75
Frequency of Replacement of Surgical Mask (Total Responses - 398)		
Response	**Percentage**	**Number of Respondents**
Daily	26.9	107
After 3 days	14.1	56
Weekly	6.5	26
Reuse	2.8	11
Don't use a surgical mask	49.7	198
Frequency of Replacement of N95 Mask (Total Mask - 386)		
Response	**Percentage**	**Number of Respondents**
Daily	4.7	18
Once in 3 days	7.5	29
Weekly	13.7	53
After 2 weeks	10.9	42
Don't use n95 mask	63.2	244
Any Health Issues Faced After Using Face Mask (Total Responses - 477)		
Response	**Percentage**	**Number of Respondents**
Yes	10.4	50
No	74.6	356
I don't know	6.0	29
Maybe	7.5	36
I don't use a mask	1.3	6
Health Issues Faced (Total Responses - 442)		

(Table 5) cont.....

Prevention of COVID-19 using Face Mask (Total Responses - 491)		
Response	**Percentage**	**Number of Respondents**
Breathing issues	25.6	113
Skin rashes	11.8	52
Itching	11.3	50
Ear pain	19.7	87
Other issues	4.3	19
No health issues	56.3	249

CONCLUDING REMARKS

Every crisis, like the current pandemic has a different impact on women than men, owing to patriarchal norms. To emerge stronger from the current scenario, policies, and tailor-made actions targeted exclusively at women are needed. Communication campaigns must be initiated so that women get first-hand information about disease prevention. Educational and vocational training must be started for women to make them find pathways to employment. The case study presented in the chapter showed that despite the discrimination suffered by the women, including the additional workload at home, they were found to be concerned for their health and well-being, which may be attributed to their educational background and the urban set-up they lived in. The survey highlighted that women could utilize the isolation period to address self-care. They were also aware of the preventive measures they should use to avert catching the COVID-19 infection.

CONSENT FOR PUBLICATION

Not applicable.

CONFLICT OF INTEREST

The authors declare no conflict of interest, financial or otherwise.

ACKNOWLEDGEMENT

Declared none.

REFERENCES

[1] Connor J, Madhavan S, Mokashi M, *et al.* Health risks and outcomes that disproportionately affect women during the Covid-19 pandemic: A review. Soc Sci Med 2020; 266: 113364. [http://dx.doi.org/10.1016/j.socscimed.2020.113364] [PMID: 32950924]

[2] Power K. The COVID-19 pandemic has increased the care burden of women and families.

Sustainability: Science. Practice and Policy 2020; 16(1): 67-73. [http://dx.doi.org/10.1080/15487733.2020.1776561]

[3] Springer KW, Mager Stellman J, Jordan-Young RM. Beyond a catalogue of differences: A theoretical frame and good practice guidelines for researching sex/gender in human health. Soc Sci Med 2012; 74(11): 1817-24. [http://dx.doi.org/10.1016/j.socscimed.2011.05.033] [PMID: 21724313]

[4] CDC health disparities and inequalities report -United States, 2013. MMWR Morb Mortal Wkly Rep 2013; 62 (Suppl. 3): 85-154.

[5] Mehta LS, Beckie TM, DeVon HA, *et al.* Acute myocardial infarction in women. Circulation 2016; 133(9): 916-47. [http://dx.doi.org/10.1161/CIR.0000000000000351] [PMID: 26811316]

[6] Rich-Edwards JW, Kaiser UB, Chen GL, Manson JE, Goldstein JM. Sex and gender differences research design for basic, clinical, and population studies: essentials for investigators. Endocr Rev 2018; 39(4): 424-39. [http://dx.doi.org/10.1210/er.2017-00246] [PMID: 29668873]

[7] https://www.worldometers.info/coronavirus/

[8] Harapan H, Itoh N, Yufika A, *et al.* Coronavirus disease 2019 (COVID-19): A literature review. J Infect Public Health 2020; 13(5): 667-73. [http://dx.doi.org/10.1016/j.jiph.2020.03.019] [PMID: 32340833]

[9] Nelson BW, Pettitt A, Flannery JE, Allen NB. Rapid assessment of psychological and epidemiological correlates of COVID-19 concern, financial strain, and health-related behavior change in a large online sample. PLoS One 2020; 15(11): e0241990. [http://dx.doi.org/10.1371/journal.pone.0241990] [PMID: 33175882]

[10] Cutler DM, Summers LH. The COVID-19 Pandemic and the $16 Trillion Virus. JAMA 2020; 324(15): 1495-6. [http://dx.doi.org/10.1001/jama.2020.19759] [PMID: 33044484]

[11] Wang C, Pan R, Wan X, *et al.* Immediate Psychological Responses and Associated Factors during the Initial Stage of the 2019 Coronavirus Disease (COVID-19) Epidemic among the General Population in China. Int J Environ Res Public Health 2020; 17(5): 1729. [http://dx.doi.org/10.3390/ijerph17051729] [PMID: 32155789]

[12] Huntley BJF, Huntley ES, Di Mascio D, Chen T, Berghella V, Chauhan SP. Rates of Maternal and Perinatal Mortality and Vertical Transmission in Pregnancies Complicated by Severe Acute Respiratory Syndrome Coronavirus 2 (SARS-Co-V-2) Infection. Obstet Gynecol 2020; 136(2): 303-12. [http://dx.doi.org/10.1097/AOG.0000000000004010] [PMID: 32516273]

[13] https://reliefweb.int/sites/reliefweb.int/files/resources/policy-brief-the-impact-of-covid-19--n-women-en.pdf

[14] https://www.theguardian.com/ world/2020/may/14/japan-suicides-fall-sharply-as-covid-

[15] https://www.studyfinds.org/quarantıne-qualıty-tıme-4-ın-5-parentssay-coronavirus-loc-down-has-brought-family-closertogether/

[16] https://www.unwomen.org/en/news/stories/2020/4/press-releasewomen-leaders-virtual-roundtab-e-on-covid-19

[17] https://leanin.org/article/the-coronavirus-is-a-financialcrisis-

[18] https://www.nytimes.com/2020/04/23/health/ coronavirus-measles-vaccines.html

[19] The indirect impact of COVID-19 on women Lockdown measures and school closures affect girls and women differently across the world and may have long-term negative consequences. Talha Burki reports.

[20] COVID-19 has "devastating" effect on women and girls Natalia Kanem, executive director of the UN Population Fund, is among experts warning about disrupted health services and a surge in gender-based violence. Sophie Cousins reports.

[21] Rafferty J, Mattson G, Earls MF, Yogman MW. Incorporating recognition and management of perinatal depression into pediatric practice. Pediatrics 2019; 143(1): e20183260. [http://dx.doi.org/10.1542/peds.2018-3260] [PMID: 30559118]

[22] Pieh C, Budimir S, Probst T. The effect of age, gender, income, work, and physical activity on mental health during coronavirus disease (COVID-19) lockdown in Austria. J Psychosom Res 2020; 136: 110186. [http://dx.doi.org/10.1016/j.jpsychores.2020.110186] [PMID: 32682159]

[23] Feinstein RE, Kotara S, Jones B, Shanor D, Nemeroff CB. A health care workers mental health crisis line in the age of COVID-19. Depress Anxiety 2020; 37(8): 822-6. [http://dx.doi.org/10.1002/da.23073] [PMID: 32667106]

[24] Liu N, Zhang F, Wei C, *et al.* Prevalence and predictors of PTSS during COVID-19 outbreak in China hardest-hit areas: Gender differences matter. Psychiatry Res 2020; 287: 112921. [http://dx.doi.org/10.1016/j.psychres.2020.112921] [PMID: 32240896]

[25] Manteuffel M, Williams S, Chen W, Verbrugge RR, Pittman DG, Steinkellner A. Influence of patient sex and gender on medication use, adherence, and prescribing alignment with guidelines. J Womens Health (Larchmt) 2014; 23(2): 112-9. [http://dx.doi.org/10.1089/jwh.2012.3972] [PMID: 24206025]

[26] United Nations Population Fund, 2020. Impact of the COVID-19 Pandemic on family Planning and ending gender-based violence, female genital Mutilation and child marriage (UNFPA interim technical note).

[27] Miller E, McCaw B. Intimate partner violence. N Engl J Med 2019; 380(9): 850-7. [http://dx.doi.org/10.1056/NEJMra1807166] [PMID: 30811911]

[28] Evans ML, Qasba N, Shah Arora K. COVID-19 highlights the policy barriers and complexities of postpartum sterilization. Contraception 2021; 103(1): 3-5. [http://dx.doi.org/10.1016/j.contraception.2020.10.006] [PMID: 33068611]

[29] Hanage WP, Testa C, Chen JT, *et al.* COVID-19: US federal accountability for entry, spread, and inequities—lessons for the future. Eur J Epidemiol 2020; 35(11): 995-1006. [http://dx.doi.org/10.1007/s10654-020-00689-2] [PMID: 33136249]

[30] Dalgard OS, Dowrick C, Lehtinen V, *et al.* Negative life events, social support and gender difference in depression. Soc Psychiatry Psychiatr Epidemiol 2006; 41(6): 444-51. [http://dx.doi.org/10.1007/s00127-006-0051-5] [PMID: 16572275]

[31] https://www.wfp.org/news/covid-19-will-double-number-people-facing-foodcrisesunless-swi-t-action-taken

[32] http://www.unwomen.org/en/news/in-focus/commissiononthe-status-of-women-2012/facts-and

[33] Wu Z, McGoogan JM. Characteristics of and important lessons from the coronavirus disease 2019 (COVID-19) outbreak in China: Summary of a report of 72314 cases from the chinese center for disease control and prevention. JAMA 2020; 323(13): 1239-42. [http://dx.doi.org/10.1001/jama.2020.2648] [PMID: 32091533]

[34] Naja F, Hamadeh R. Nutrition amid the COVID-19 pandemic: a multi-level framework for action. Eur J Clin Nutr 2020; 74(8): 1117-21. [http://dx.doi.org/10.1038/s41430-020-0634-3] [PMID: 32313188]

[35] Fernández-Quintela A, Milton-Laskibar I, Trepiana J, *et al.* Key Aspects in Nutritional Management of COVID-19 Patients. J Clin Med 2020; 9(8): 2589. [http://dx.doi.org/10.3390/jcm9082589] [PMID: 32785121]

[36] https://data.unwomen.org/resources/surveys-show-covid-19-hasgendered-

[37] 2016.http://uis.unesco.org/en/country/in

[38] Prochaska JO, Velicer WF. The transtheoretical model of health behavior change. Am J Health Promot 1997; 12(1): 38-48.
[http://dx.doi.org/10.4278/0890-1171-12.1.38] [PMID: 10170434]

[39] Mościcka P, Chróst N, Terlikowski R, Przylipiak M, Wołosik K, Przylipiak A. Hygienic and cosmetic care habits in polish women during COVID-19 pandemic. J Cosmet Dermatol 2020; 19(8): 1840-5.
[http://dx.doi.org/10.1111/jocd.13539] [PMID: 32573966]

[40] Schneider S, May M, Stone AA. Careless responding in internet-based quality of life assessments. Qual Life Res 2018; 27(4): 1077-88.
[http://dx.doi.org/10.1007/s11136-017-1767-2] [PMID: 29248996]

CHAPTER 5

Vaccination Hesitancy and Adaptation with Particular Emphasis on Women

Tahmeena Khan[1], **Alfred J. Lawrence**[2,*], **Amos Nascimento**[3] and **Rohan Srivastava**[1]

[1] *Integral University, Lucknow, India*

[2] *Department of Chemistry, Isabella Thoburn College, Lucknow-226007, Uttar Pradesh, India*

[3] *University of Washington, Tacoma/Seattle, USA*

Abstract: The novel beta-coronavirus SARS-CoV-2 (COVID-19) emerged in 2019 in Wuhan from bats and later caused inter-human transmission. India is one of the worst-hit countries, where two million casualties have taken place during the second wave of the pandemic. The year 2021 witnessed the more deadly form of the virus. At the same time, there was remarkable progress in vaccine development resulting in the approval of a few vaccines by the governments. The process of COVID-19 vaccination has kickstarted in many countries. The general attitude towards acceptance of the vaccine has been reported in countries like the USA and Jordan. Very few studies have reported the understanding and hesitation regarding the vaccination among the Indian population, and the present study is an attempt to highlight the general mindset, acceptance, misconceptions and awareness regarding the COVID-19 vaccination from the Indian perspective. Being one of the worst-hit countries in terms of COVID-19, it is important to identify the barriers holding the Indian population back from getting vaccinated. This study was done as a questionnaire survey aimed at knowing the general apprehension, and thoughts of the public regarding the vaccination with 308 respondents, precisely of Indian origin. 58.8% (n=181) respondents were non-vaccinated. 45.2% (n=95) respondents reported that their respective employers made vaccination compulsory. 51.5% (n=120) felt that the vaccine is 60-80% safe. The results may be used by the public health authorities to identify the priority group and the barriers holding people back from vaccination.

Keywords: Acceptance, Concerns, COVID-19, Hesitation, Immunity, India, Longevity, Misconception, Side Effects, Vaccination.

* **Corresponding author Alfred J. Lawrence:** Department of Chemistry, Isabella Thoburn College, Lucknow-226007, Uttar Pradesh, India: E-mail: Alfred_lawrence@yahoo.com

INTRODUCTION

The coronavirus was first identified in 1965 in studies developed by Tyrrell and Bynoe, who identified a virus that they named B814 [1]. Since then, a morphological similarity was noticed between transmissible cases of ovine bronchitis, hepatitis in rodents and swine gastroenteritis virus. Due to the fact that, morphologically, this type of virus had external projections in the form of a crown, this new group was named "corona virus." After decades of research, evidence showed that the coronavirus was responsible for respiratory diseases in several animal species, including rodents, sheep, cattle and swine, as well as cats and dogs [2]. Over time, it was discovered that respiratory diseases in humans, especially children.

These correlations remained somewhat unnoticed by the larger public until 2003, when the coronavirus was identified as the cause of a new disease, Severe Acute Respiratory Syndrome (SARS), that emerged in southern China and spread throughout the world quickly. Infectious cases emerged in 29 countries in Asia, the Americas, and Europe, reaching about 8,000 cases and almost 800 deaths. This was followed by several other virological discoveries in Hong Kong (China), Amsterdam (Netherlands), and New Haven (United States) – the latter being called "New Have Coronavirus (HCoV-NH) – as well as international epidemic cases such as the avian flu and swine flu (H1N1) [3]. With technological advances, it was possible to not only carry out serological tests but also to carry out the genetic sequencing of the various types of this virus. In this process, it was concluded that the virus was transmissible not only through the zoonotic route, but also through human vectors. These and other developments in coronavirology led to new hypotheses about the possibility of new epidemics [4].

The novel beta-coronavirus SARS-CoV-2 and the novel coronavirus disease 2019 (COVID-19) emerged in the year 2019 in Wuhan, China, as a result of high-impact zoonoses traced back to bats (order Chiroptera) and viral diseases identified earlier in Southern China [5, 6]. While studies were being carried out to identify its exact origination, COVID-19 reached 188 countries and 25 territories globally, despite the best efforts of governments and the World Health Organization (WHO) [7], due to the high transmission ability of the virus [7]. As the coronavirus is responsible for various respiratory diseases, it spreads by the inhalation of aerosols and through interpersonal contact. While various new vaccines have been developed in different countries, no concrete medicinal cure has been found to date. Therefore, physical distancing, personal hygiene, washing of hands and sanitization with 70% alcohol-based sanitizer have been suggested as precautionary measures to keep the infection at bay [8]. Those suffering from any other co-morbid conditions are at greater risk of getting infected and having severe symptoms. The incubation period of the virus is said to be of 5.1 days [9]. The symptoms of the disease include fever, dry cough, shortness of breath, chills and dysentery [9].

Coronaviruses are pleomorphic and enveloped with peculiar projections protruding from their surface consisting of S protein. The genome of the novel coronavirus is transcribed in 10 open reading frames (ORFs), translating into a polyprotein processing into 16 non-structural proteins (NSPs) [10]. The non-structural proteins help in genome replication, capping, tailing, which are necessary for the maintenance of the virus [11]. The SARS-CoV-2 virus also contains four structural proteins, namely spike (S), nucleocapsid (N), envelope (E), and membrane (M) proteins encoded by the 3-end of the viral genome [12]. Amongst the four structural proteins, the S glycoprotein, being a multi-functional trans-membrane protein, has an important role in viral attachment and its entry into the host cell [12]. The S protein consists of S1 and S2 subunits splitting into different functional domains. The S1 subunits consist of two domains viz. N-terminal Domain (NTD) and Receptor Binding Domain (RBD), consisting of conserved receptor binding motif (RBM) [13]. Immunotherapy is one of the most efficient methods used for the cure of different contagious diseases and cancer. The technique included the activation of the immune system to enhance the immune response [14]. The COVID-19 vaccines are usually targeted with an aim to generate S protein-neutralizing antibodies. Studies have found almost no cross-neutralization between the sera of SARS-CoV and SARS-CoV-2, showing that those recovering from one infection are not necessarily safe from the other [15]. More than five thousand full-length genomes of SARs-CoV-2 have been derived from different nations, which delineate the polymorphisms in S and other proteins of the virus responsible for vaccine development. Most of the vaccines developed against COVID-19 have been using S-protein [16]. Multiple nations across the globe have initiated vaccination under emergency authorization, and US FDA has approved Pfizer and Moderna, whereas the UK regulatory bodies have approved three vaccines *viz*., Pfizer, AstraZeneca and Moderna based on the efficacy and safety data obtained from phase III trials. India being one of the worst-hit countries, has approved two vaccines and initiated its largest vaccination drive initially from frontline workers and older adults. Pune-based Serum Institute's Covishield and Hyderabad-based Bharat Biotech's Covaxin have been approved by the Indian government. Covishield has passed the phase III trials, whereas Covaxin is still undergoing phase III trial [17]. The approved vaccines are based on either inactivated or active attenuated viruses, protein-sub units, virus-like particles (VLP), replicating and non-replicating viral vectors, DNA, RNA, and nano-particles, *etc*., showing their own exclusive properties [18]. To augment the immunogenicity, various adjuvant techniques like AS03 (GSK), MF-59 (Novartis), CpG 1018 (Dynavax), *etc*., are also available for the effective development of the vaccine [19]. Reverse vaccinology (RV) is a recent methodology that identifies the promising vaccine candidate by applying bioinformatics and computational approach for the analysis of the pathogen genome. The two design strategies for vaccine development include the usage of the whole virus or genetically engineered vaccine antigens delivered through different designs. The whole virus vaccines include inactivated or live attenuated vaccines [20]. The two live attenuated SARS vaccines mutated the exoribonuclease and enveloped protein to diminish the virulence and replication capability of the virus. The whole virus vaccines lead to a strong immune response and protect against infections. Genetically engineered vaccines targeting specific coronavirus proteins are seldom used to improve safety and effectiveness. The coronavirus antigens such as S protein, N protein, and M protein can be delivered as recombinant DNA vaccine and viral vector vaccine. The Pfizer and Moderna vaccines developed in the United States have an efficiency of more than 90%, whereas the AstraZeneca vaccine, developed in the UK, has an efficacy rate of 62% after the two doses. In India, two main vaccines have been developed and applied: Covishield and Covaxin. Covishield, an Indian version of AstraZeneca, is a recombinant adenovirus vaccine developed by the use of S glycoprotein and produced with the tissue plasminogen activator (tPA) as the preferred vaccine [21]. Covaxin, made by Bharat Biotech, is developed with Whole-Virion Inactivated Vero Cell-derived technology and contains an inactivated virus. Although the data clearly indicates that the vaccines are safe, the general public is still hesitant and reluctant to get vaccinated and has serious safety concerns. This study was done as a questionnaire survey aimed at knowing the general apprehension and thoughts of the public regarding the COVID-19 vaccination.

A QUESTIONNAIRE-BASED STUDY

The questionnaire was prepared as a Google form and sent electronically to the respondents above 18 years of age between 1st May- 1st September, 2021. The questionnaire was circulated through postgraduate students on different WhatsApp groups. To facilitate snowball sampling, the link of the questionnaire was also shared on different social media platforms. The questions were included based on a literature survey and previous studies and approved by experts. The survey was self-administered on a voluntary basis, and all the personal information of the respondents was kept confidential. Clear instructions were given in the form. The responses were downloaded from the Google form. Data were collected according to Helsinki's declaration. The first section of the questionnaire included demographic information. The second section collected information about the awareness related to COVID-19 vaccine and the willingness to get vaccinated. Section three included questions about the safety concerns, and apprehensions related to the side effects and efficiency of the vaccine. The last section evaluated their knowledge about COVID-19 in relation to immunity and the effect of the vaccine. The questionnaire was posted on social media sites to facilitate snowball sampling. Not all the questions were kept mandatory to keep the interest of the respondent intact. The data was tabulated in MS Excel.

RESULTS AND DISCUSSION

Demographic Details

Demographic characteristics like age group, marital status, area of living, religion and number of family members are important and crucial for choice-making and make one understands the background features of the respondents well. Demographic details are also important to identify the priority groups on the basis of their age and the region they belong to. 98.5% (n=303) respondents were Indian nationals out of which 80.5% (n=248) were females. Majority of the respondents (n=215) belonged to 18-30 age group bracket (Table **1**) and belonged to urban households. The demographic details may help public health officials ensure the efficient and equitable distribution of the vaccine to the high priority groups more susceptible to catching infection.

COVID-19 Vaccine Awareness

Of the total responses, 58.8% (n=181) did not receive their vaccination dose. However, vaccination is the only way to contain the spread of the virus. 75% (n=102) had a Covishield jab, whereas 16.2% (n=22) opted for Bharat Biotech-made Covaxin. Covishield was the most sought-after vaccine, as declared by 46.4% (n=143) respondents. It is a recombinant adenovirus vaccine developed by the use of S glycoprotein and produced with the tissue plasminogen activator (tPA). 82.4% (n=168) people were positive about getting vaccinated and planned to get their dose depending upon the availability of the vaccine (Table **2**). Month-wise vaccination is reported in (Fig. **1**). It is important to identify the population's intentions to get vaccinated and the hurdles to enhancing the rate of vaccination [22]. Although the number of vaccinated respondents at the time of filling out the questionnaire was low, either their spouse or parents had been vaccinated, as shown by 3.1% (n=225) respondents. Among the vaccinated individuals, 45.2% (n=95) declared that their respective employers made vaccination compulsory for the employees (Table **2**). 73% (n=142) respondents decided for themselves whether to get vaccinated. Vaccine approval may lead to an end of the pandemic by creating herd immunity [23], which is anticipated to be between 50%-67%. But the skeptical attitude of people may deter them from achieving such a huge task. WHO has defined vaccine hesitancy as "delay in acceptance or refusal of vaccination despite the availability of vaccination services" [24]. The acceptability depends upon confidence, convenience and complacency [25]. Skepticism has been demonstrated in a survey conducted in the US, where 50% of Americans were found to be more acceptable towards a vaccine, 30% were unsure, while 20% did not give their consent the vaccine [26]. In another survey-based study with adult Americans, 58% showed their inclination to get vaccinated; on the other hand, 32% were reluctant or unsure, and 11% did not intend to be vaccinated [27]. One more survey-based study showed that 67% of Americans may accept the vaccine upon recommendation, although there were significant demographic differences in vaccine acceptance [28].

Table 1. Demographic Details.

Gender of the Respondents, Total Responses=308		
Gender	**Respondents**	**Percentage**
Male	60	19.5
Female	248	80.5
Others	0	0
Country of Residence, Total Responses =308		
Country	**Respondents**	**Percentage**
India	303	98.5
Switzerland	2	0.6
United States	3	1
Age Group, Total Responses=301		
Age Group	**Respondents**	**Percentage**
18-30	215	71.4
30-40	19	6.3
40-50	26	8.6
Above 50	29	9.6
Above 55	5	1.7
30-35	4	1.3
45-55	2	0.7
35-45	1	0.3

Table 2. COVID-19 Awareness.

Have you Received a COVID-19 Vaccine?, Total Responses=308		
	Respondents	**Percentage**
Yes	127	41.2

(Table 2) cont.....

Have you Received a COVID-19 Vaccine?, Total Responses=308		
No	181	58.8
If Yes, Then Which Vaccine you Have Received?, Total Responses=136		
Vaccine	**Respondents**	**Percentage**
Covaxin	22	16.2
Covishield	102	75
Pfizer Biontech	5	3.7
Sinopharm	0	0
Moderna	4	2.9
Sputnik	1	0.7
Oxfard - astrazeneca	1	0.7
Johnson-johnson	1	0.7
Coronavac	1	0.7
If No, Then Do You Plan To Get Vaccinated, Total Responses= 204		
Response	**Respondents**	**Percentage**
Yes	168	82.4
No	12	5.9
Maybe	24	11.8
You Opted For Vaccination After, Total Responses=194		
Response	**Respondents**	**Percentage**
Instructions of government	40	20.6
Instructions of your employer	6	3.1
Decided for yourself	142	73.2
Under family pressure	6	3.1
Are You Ready To Get Vaccinated If Provided By Your Employer? Total Responses= 210		
Response	**Respondents**	**Percentage**
Yes	95	45.2
No	71	33.8
Maybe	44	21
Have Your Spouse, Parents Been Vaccinated?, Total Responses= 308		
Response	**Respondents**	**Percentage**
Yes	225	73.1%
No	83	26.9%
If Yes, Who Among Them Got Vaccinated?, Total Responses= 222		
Response	**Respondents**	**Percentage**

(Table 2) cont.....

Have you Received a COVID-19 Vaccine?, Total Responses=308		
Mother	21	9.5
Father	102	45.9
Wife	11	5
Husband	18	8.1
All	70	31.5

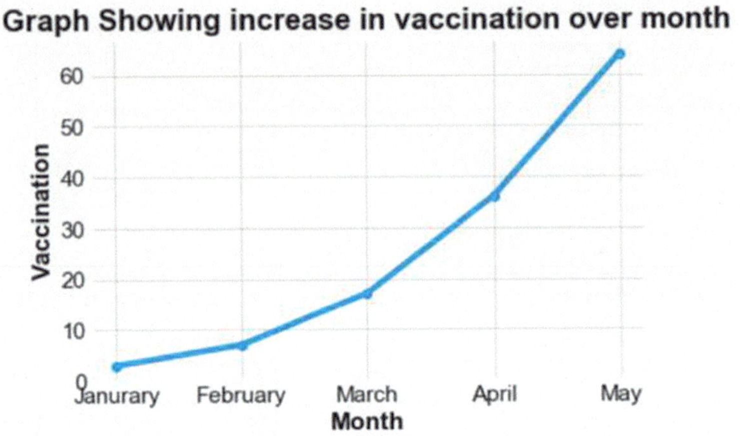

Fig. (1). Month in which vaccination was done.

Safety Concerns Related to Vaccination

When a person goes for vaccination, there are certain apprehensions and concerns involved. 27.3% (n=84) respondents expressed their confusion over choosing the appropriate vaccine for themselves among all the available options, whereas, 16.2% (n=50) had an apprehension regarding the side effects. Safety concerns (4.5%) and fear of catching COVID infection after vaccination (4.9%) were other reported concerns (Fig. **2**). Questions usually arise on the efficiency of a newly developed vaccine which could be lessened when the vaccine is easily available and its success rate increases [28]. A recent study has shown that people are apprehensive of the fact that the vaccine has been approved in haste owing to political pressure. Once the factors leading to apprehension are identified, the government may organize awareness campaigns to increase the rate of vaccination. A significant number of respondents felt that they might fall into the high-risk category to catch COVID infection. The perceived fear may channel vaccination hesitancy [29]. Therefore consciousness is an essential parameter for improving willingness. Post-vaccination symptoms were most commonly reported by females (54%, n=106), which usually occurred after 10-12 h of dosage (65.2%, n=131). Fever (36.7%, n=72) and fatigue/tiredness (21.4%, n=42) were the most common and prominent side effects experienced after vaccination. In the majority of the cases (27%, n=43), the symptoms persisted for 24 h after dosage (Fig. **3**) whereas, 23.9% (n=38) respondents experienced the side effects 48 h after dosage. Low immunity was cited by 49% (n=48) respondents as a probable cause to catch COVID infection. Among the respondents, 30.2% (n=93) thought that the duration of protection is the major reason associated with people not opting for vaccination whereas 29.5% (n=91) thought that the fear associated with long-term complications is holding people back from getting vaccinated (Table **3**). Common reasons of avoiding vaccines are given in (Fig. **4**). Mainly all vaccines challenge the immune system leading to an increase in the inflammatory markers within a few hours of the administration of vaccine. The innate immune response is responsible for producing side effects such as fever, fatigue, malaise and irritability. The inflammatory response generally lasts a few days, and in exceptional cases, particularly in individuals with high-stress levels, it can last longer [30]. The adaptive immune system mounts the second spike of the immune response targeting particular vaccine components and takes a longer time to act. The vaccines are designed in such a manner that the adaptive immune response system develops a long-term memory of the viral or bacterial components and responds instantly when it comes in contact with the actual pathogen [31].

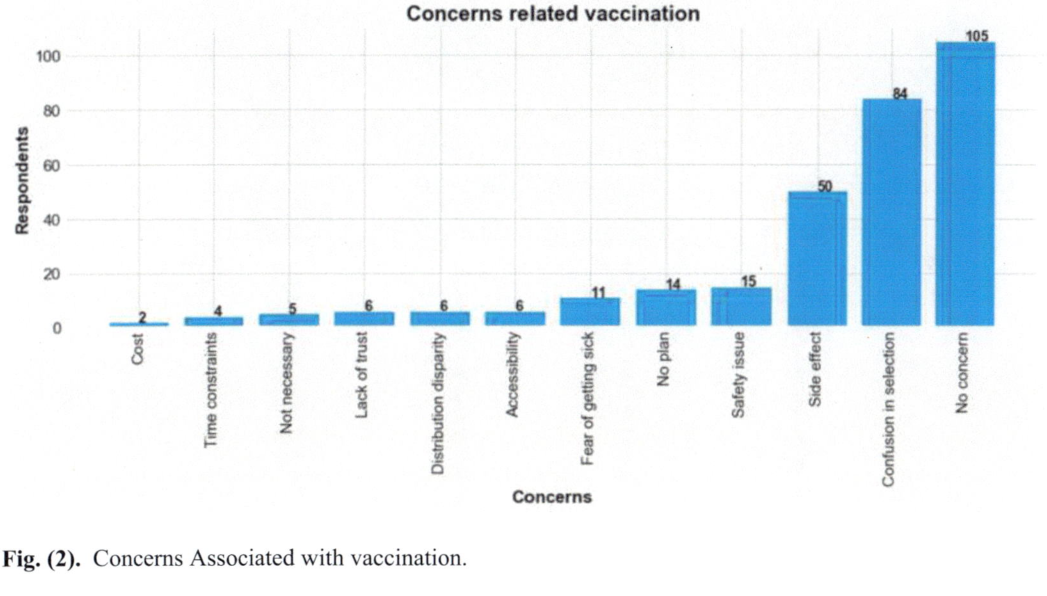

Fig. (2). Concerns Associated with vaccination.

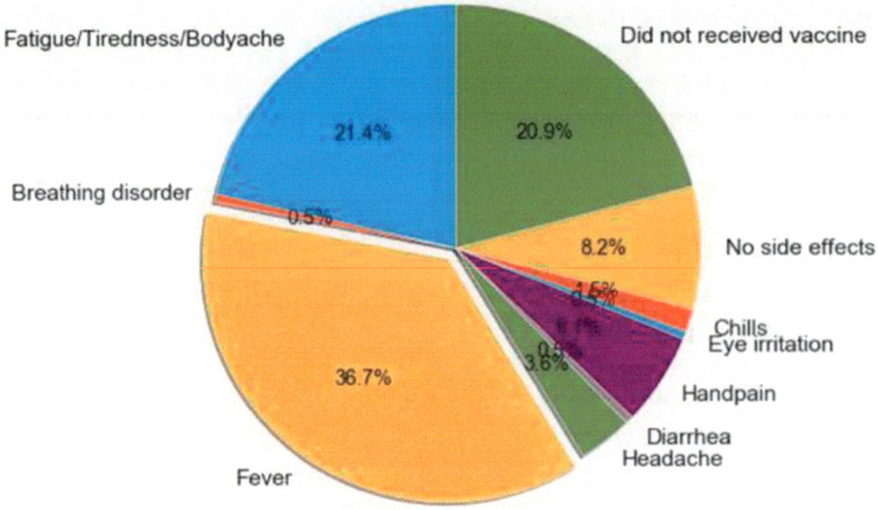

Fig. (3). Side effects observed after vaccination.

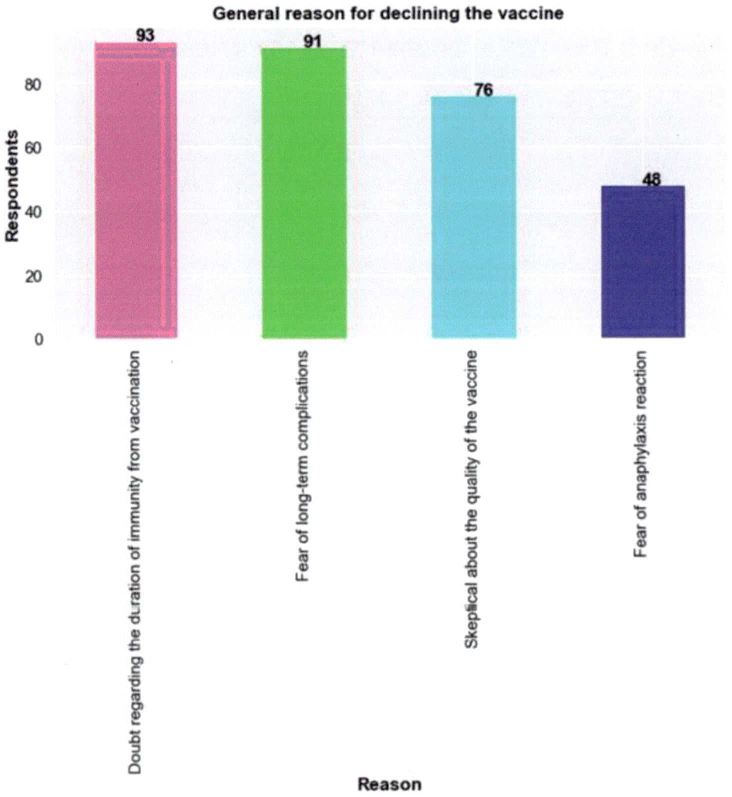

Fig. (4). Common reason for avoiding vaccination.

Misconceptions and Disbeliefs

To assess the misconceptions related to the COVID-19 vaccination, this section was included. 51.5% (n=120) respondents felt that the vaccine is 60-80% safe 42.12% (n=99) respondents felt that pregnant or breastfeeding mothers must not take the vaccine shot. Some of them felt that people prone to any allergy or small children under 18 should also avoid vaccine. 87% (n=268) respondents reported that even if the side effects are not experienced after vaccination, it still does not mean that the vaccine is not working. 82.8% (n=255) respondents trusted the quality of vaccine the government is providing and 57.6% (n=99) felt that their immunity would last long after getting vaccinated, and 90.2% (n=203) respondents did not feel that their natural antibodies would be destroyed after getting the vaccination done and 46.5% (n=99) also felt that the vaccine may also shield them against other viruses as well. The antibody levels may be an important indicator of lasting immunity [32]. It is an important marker to assess the protection against SARS-CoV-2 [33]. Antibody levels may remain high even after six months of getting infected [32], but still, it is not the only marker to assess the level of protection. It was quite interesting to find that the seriousness related to the vaccination was not associated with the COVID-19 infection. Most of the respondents who did not catch COVID infection were willing to take the vaccine. The information related to the misconceptions and misbeliefs and general knowledge regarding the vaccination is given in Tables **4 and 5**. The longevity and effectiveness of the vaccine, as reported by the respondents, are given in (Fig. **5**).

Table 3. Safety concerns and risk assessment.

How Safe is COVID-19 Vaccine? Total Responses=91		
Response	**Respondents**	**Percentage**
20-40%	9	3.9
40-60%	31	13.3
60-80%	120	51.5
80-100%	73	31.3
Who should Not Take The COVID-19 Vaccine? Total Responses =235		
Response	**Respondents**	**Percentage**
People prone to some allergy	55	23.4
Small children (under 18)	76	32.3
People above 70 years of age	5	2.1
Pregnant and/or breastfeeding mothers	99	42.1
Does The Lack Of Side Effects Mean That The Vaccine Is Not Working? Total Responses=308		

(Table 3) cont.....

Response	Respondents	Percentage
Yes	40	13
No	268	87
Do You Trust Government With The Quality Of The Vaccine Being Provided? Total Responses= 308		
Response	**Respondents**	**Percentage**
Yes	255	82.8
No	53	17.2
Are You Feeling Psychologically More Positive After Taking The Vaccine Shot? Total Responses=162		
Response	**Respondents**	**Percentage**
Yes	130	80.2
No	32	19.8
Does Immunity After Getting Covid-19 Vaccine? Total Responses=172		
Response	**Respondents**	**Percentage**
Yes	99	57.6
No	73	42.4
Will Natural Antibodies Be Destroyed After Vaccination? Total Responses =225		
Response	**Respondents**	**Percentage**
Yes	22	9.8
No	203	90.2
Can Covid-19 Vaccine Give Immunity Against Other Viruses As Well? Total Responses = 213		
Response	**Respondents**	**Percentage**
Yes	114	53.5
No	99	46.5
Did You Quarantine Yourself After Getting Vaccine? Total Responses 163		
Response	**Respondents**	**Percentage**
Yes	65	39.9
No	98	60.1
Should Pain Reliever Be Taken Pre Or Post Vaccination? Total Responses = 211		
Response	**Respondents**	**Percentage**
Yes	42	19.9%
No	67	31.8%
Maybe	102	48.3%
Any Lab Tests Required Before Vaccination? Total Responses= 189		
Response	**Respondents**	**Percentage**
Yes	34	18%

(Table 3) cont.....

No	155	82%
If Yes, These Prominently Include, Total Responses=58		
Test	**Respondents**	**Percentage**
Routine blood test	25	43.1%
Ecgs	4	6.9%
Ultrasounds	1	1.7%
Other medical screening tests	28	48.3%

Table 4. COVID-19 beliefs and misconceptions.

You are in a High-Risk Category to Catch COVID-19 Infection?, Total Responses= 308		
Response	**Respondents**	**Percentage**
Yes	61	19.8
No	168	54.5
Maybe	79	25.6
If Yes, Then Why?, Total Responses=98		
Response	**Respondents**	**Percentage**
Because You Are A Health Worker	14	14.3
Because You Have Other Co-Morbidities	24	24.5
Because You Have A Low Immunity	48	49
Because You Have Already Contracted covid-19 Infection	12	12.2
Post Vaccination Symptoms are more Prominent in, Total Responses=195		
Gender	**Respondents**	**Percentage**
Males	62	31.8
Females	106	54.4
Others	27	13.8
Are Covid Vaccine Side Effects Immediate?, Total Responses=253		
Response	**Respondents**	**Percentage**
Yes	41	16.2
No	127	50.2
Maybe	85	33.6

(Table 4) cont.....

If Not Immediate, After How Long The Post Vaccination Symptoms Appeared?, Total Responses=201		
Duration	**Respondents**	**Percentage**
10 -12 h of Dosage	131	65.2
24 h of Dosage	39	19.4
After 24 h Of Dosage	31	15.4
If You Have Got Vaccinated, Then For How Long The Post Vaccination Symptoms Persisted? Total Responses= 159		
Duration	**Respondents**	**Percentage**
12 h After Dosage	35	22
24 h After Dosage	43	27
48 h After Dosage	38	23.9
More Than 48 h	13	8.2
No Symptoms	30	18.9

Table 5. COVID-19 infection Vs COVID-19 Vaccine.

Does A Person Affected With Covid-19 Recommended To Take Vaccine?, Total Responses= 308		
Response	**Respondents**	**Percentage**
Yes	226	73.4
No	82	26.6
If Yes, After How Many Days Vaccination Should Be Done? Total Responses= 213		
Response	**Respondents**	**Percentage**
Within 7 days	6	2.8
After 7 days	13	6.1
After 1 month	51	23.9
After more than 1 month	132	62
After 4 months	5	3.2
After 2 months	3	1.4
After 3 Months	3	1.4
Can One Take First Dose Of One Vaccine And Second Dose Of Other? Total Responses=308		
Response	**Respondents**	**Percentage**
Yes	38	12.3
No	270	87.7
Did You Take Vaccine After Contracting COVID-19? Total Responses=308		
Response	**Respondents**	**Percentage**
Yes	26	8.4

(Table 5) cont.....

No	128	41.6
Did not get vaccinated	154	50%
Did You Contract Covid Infection Again, After Taking The Vaccine Shots?		
TOTAL RESPONSES=308		
	Respondents	**Percentage**
Yes	15	4.9
No	136	44.2
Did not get vaccinated	157	51
After How Many Days, The Second Dose Of Covid-19 Vaccine Was Taken? Total Responses=176		
Duration	**Respondents**	**Percentage**
10 days	1	0.6
20 days	9	5.1
30 days	28	15.9
40 days	11	6.3
More than 40 days	14	8
Have not taken second dose yet	113	64.2

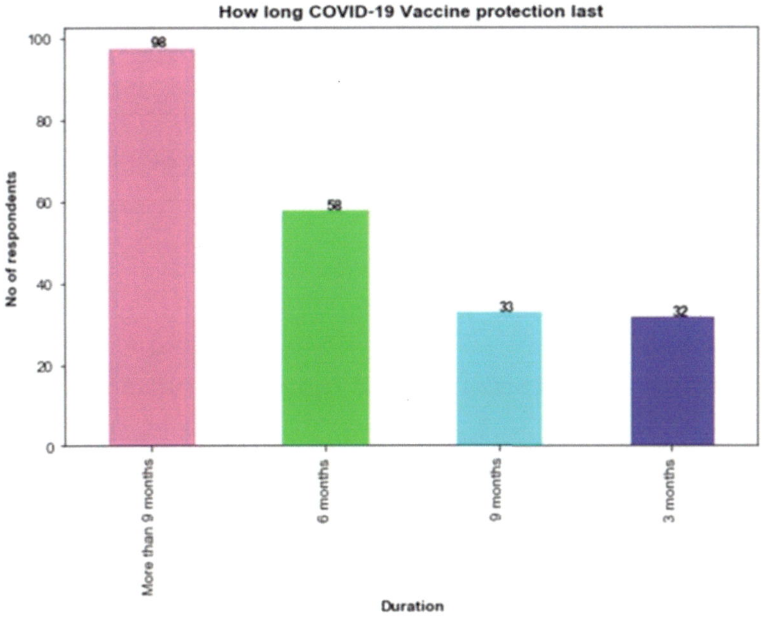

Fig. (5). Longevity of the effect of the vaccine.

CONCLUSION

The SARS-CoV-2 pandemic has jolted the world on multiple levels. Scientists across the world have come up with a solution in the form of a vaccine that may save from the severity of the disease. But curiosity, safety concerns and availability keep people from vaccinating. This questionnaire survey shed light on crucial aspects related to the vaccination process, primarily targeting the Indian female population. At the time of compilation of the results, 58% of the respondents were still not vaccinated. Many of them got vaccinated after being pressurized by their respective employers. On the brighter side, people were positive about getting vaccinated in the future as and when it becomes available to them. They were also aware of the fact that even after getting a COVID infection, they can still get vaccinated. They were also aware of the options available to them. The reluctance to get vaccinated was primarily due to the safety and efficacy issues and the development of any long-term complications. It is the urgent responsibility of the public health authorities to hold awareness campaigns to educate the public on the relevance of getting vaccinated in this scenario and clear off the myths and misconceptions

CONSENT FOR PUBLICATION

Not applicable.

CONFLICT OF INTEREST

The authors declare no conflict of interest, financial or otherwise.

ACKNOWLEDGEMENT

Declared none.

References

[1] Tyrrell DAJ, Bynoe ML. Cultivation of a Novel Type of Common-cold Virus in Organ Cultures. BMJ 1965; 1(5448): 1467-70. [http://dx.doi.org/10.1136/bmj.1.5448.1467] [PMID: 14288084]

[2] Machlachlan NJ, Dubovi EJ, Eds. Fenner's Veterinary Virology . (Academic Press/Elsevier), chapter 24, "Coronaviridae," 2011; pp. 394-413.

[3] de Wit E, van Doremalen N, Falzarano D, Munster VJ. SARS and MERS: recent insights into emerging coronaviruses. Nat Rev Microbiol 2016; 14(8): 523-34. [http://dx.doi.org/10.1038/nrmicro.2016.81] [PMID: 27344959]

[4] Li H, Mendelsohn E. Human-animal interactions and bat coronavirus spillover potential among rural residents in Southern China. Biosafety and Health 2019; pp. 84-90. [http://dx.doi.org/10.1016/j.bsheal.2019.10.004]

[5] Gralinsky L, Menachery V. Return of the Coronavirus: 2019 n-Cov. Viruses 2020; 12(135): 1-8. [http://dx.doi.org/10.3390/v12020135.]

[6] Shereen MA, Khan S, Kazmi A, Bashir N, Siddique R. COVID-19 infection: Emergence, transmission, and characteristics of human coronaviruses. J Adv Res 2020; 24: 91-8. [http://dx.doi.org/10.1016/j.jare.2020.03.005] [PMID: 32257431]

[7] Lai CC, Shih TP, Ko WC, Tang HJ, Hsueh PR. Severe acute respiratory syndrome coronavirus 2 (SARS-CoV-2) and coronavirus disease-2019 (COVID-19): The epidemic and the challenges. Int J Antimicrob Agents 2020; 55(3): 105924. [http://dx.doi.org/10.1016/j.ijantimicag.2020.105924] [PMID: 32081636]

[8] Chan JFW, Kok KH, Zhu Z, *et al.* Genomic characterization of the 2019 novel human-pathogenic coronavirus isolated from a patient with atypical pneumonia after visiting Wuhan. Emerg Microbes Infect 2020; 9(1): 221-36. [http://dx.doi.org/10.1080/22221751.2020.1719902] [PMID: 31987001]

[9] Lauer SA, Grantz KH, Bi Q, *et al.* The Incubation Period of Coronavirus Disease 2019 (COVID-19) From Publicly Reported Confirmed Cases: Estimation and Application. Ann Intern Med 2020; 172(9): 577-82. [http://dx.doi.org/10.7326/M20-0504] [PMID: 32150748]

[10] Yoshimoto FK. The Proteins of Severe Acute Respiratory Syndrome Coronavirus-2 (SARS CoV-2 or n-COV19), the Cause of COVID-19. Protein J 2020; 39(3): 198-216. [http://dx.doi.org/10.1007/s10930-020-09901-4] [PMID: 32447571]

[11] Silva SJR, Alves da Silva CT, Mendes RPG, Pena L. Role of nonstructural proteins in the pathogenesis of SARS□CoV□2. J Med Virol 2020; 92(9): 1427-9. [http://dx.doi.org/10.1002/jmv.25858] [PMID: 32270884]

[12] Wrapp D, Wang N, Corbett KS, *et al.* Cryo-EM structure of the 2019-nCoV spike in the prefusion conformation. Science 2020; 367(6483): 1260-3. [http://dx.doi.org/10.1126/science.abb2507] [PMID: 32075877]

[13] Jiang S, Du L, Shi Z. An emerging coronavirus causing pneumonia outbreak in Wuhan, China: calling for developing therapeutic and prophylactic strategies. Emerg Microbes Infect 2020; 9(1): 275-7. [http://dx.doi.org/10.1080/22221751.2020.1723441] [PMID: 32005086]

[14] Masihi KN. Fighting infection using immunomodulatory agents. Expert Opin Biol Ther 2001; 1(4): 641-53. [http://dx.doi.org/10.1517/14712598.1.4.641] [PMID: 11727500]

[15] Ou X, Liu Y, Lei X, *et al.* Characterization of spike glycoprotein of SARS-CoV-2 on virus entry and its immune cross-reactivity with SARS-CoV. Nat Commun 2020; 11(1): 1620. [http://dx.doi.org/10.1038/s41467-020-15562-9] [PMID: 32221306]

[16] Dhama K, Sharun K, Tiwari R, *et al.* COVID-19, an emerging coronavirus infection: advances and prospects in designing and developing vaccines, immunotherapeutics, and therapeutics. Hum Vaccin Immunother 2020; 16(6): 1232-8. [http://dx.doi.org/10.1080/21645515.2020.1735227] [PMID: 32186952]

[17] Kumar VM, Pandi-Perumal SR, Trakht I, *et al.* Strategy for COVID-19 vaccination in India: the country with the second highest population and number of cases. npj. Vaccines (Basel) 2021; 6: (60). [http://dx.doi.org/10.1038/s41541-021-00327-2]

[18] Wang N, Shang J, Jiang S, Du L. Subunit Vaccines Against Emerging Pathogenic Human Coronaviruses. Front Microbiol 2020; 11: 298. [http://dx.doi.org/10.3389/fmicb.2020.00298] [PMID: 32265848]

[19] Thanh Le T, Andreadakis Z, Kumar A, *et al.* The COVID-19 vaccine development landscape. Nat Rev Drug Discov 2020; 19(5): 305-6. [http://dx.doi.org/10.1038/d41573-020-00073-5] [PMID: 32273591]

[20] Graham RL, Becker MM, Eckerle LD, *et al.* A live, impaired-fidelity coronavirus vaccine protects in an aged, immunocompromised mouse model of lethal disease. Nat Med 2012;18(12):1820-26.

[http://dx.doi.org/10.1038/nm.2972]

[21] Al-Qerem WA, Jarab AS. COVID-19 Vaccination Acceptance and Its Associated Factors Among a Middle Eastern Population. Front Public Health 2021; 9: 632914. [http://dx.doi.org/10.3389/fpubh.2021.632914]

[22] Kreps S, Prasad S, Brownstein JS, *et al.* Factors associated with US adults' likelihood of accepting COVID-19 vaccination. JAMA Netw Open 2020; 3(10): e2025594. [http://dx.doi.org/10.1001/jamanetworkopen.2020.25594] [PMID: 33079199]

[23] Ward JK, Alleaume C, Peretti-Watel P, *et al.* The French public's attitudes to a future COVID-19 vaccine: The politicization of a public health issue. Soc Sci Med 2020; 265: 113414. [http://dx.doi.org/10.1016/j.socscimed.2020.113414] [PMID: 33038683]

[24] Neumann-Böhme S, Varghese NE, Sabat I, *et al.* Once we have it, will we use it? A European survey on willingness to be vaccinated against COVID-19. Eur J Health Econ 2020; 21(7): 977-82. [http://dx.doi.org/10.1007/s10198-020-01208-6] [PMID: 32591957]

[25] Madison AA, Shrout MR, Renna ME, Kiecolt-Glaser JK. Psychological and Behavioral Predictors of Vaccine Efficacy: Considerations for COVID-19. Perspect Psychol Sci 2021; 16(2): 191-203. [http://dx.doi.org/10.1177/1745691621989243] [PMID: 33501900]

[26] Zuo J, Dowell A, Pearce H, *et al.* Robust SARS-CoV-2-specific T-cell immunity is maintained at 6 months following primary infection. Nat Immunol 2021; 2(5): 620-6. [http://dx.doi.org/10.21203/rs.3.rs-101480/v1]

[27] Tan W, Lu Y, Zhang J, *et al.* Viral kinetics and antibody responses in patients with COVID-19. MedRxiv [http://dx.doi.org/10.1101/2020.03.24.20042382]

[28] Kaur SP, Gupta V. COVID-19 Vaccine: A comprehensive status report. Virus Res 2020; 288: 198114. [http://dx.doi.org/10.1016/j.virusres.2020.198114] [PMID: 32800805]

[29] Omer SB, Yildirim I, Forman HP. Herd Immunity and Implications for SARS-CoV-2 Control. JAMA 2020; 324(20): 2095-6. [http://dx.doi.org/10.1001/jama.2020.20892] [PMID: 33074293]

[30] Al-Mohaithef M, Padhi BK. Determinants of COVID-19 Vaccine Acceptance in Saudi Arabia: A Web-Based National Survey. J Multidiscip Healthc 2020; 13: 1657-63. [http://dx.doi.org/10.2147/JMDH.S276771] [PMID: 33262600]

[31] https://apnews.com/article/dacdc8bc428dd4df6511bfa259cfec44

[32] Fisher KA, Bloomstone SJ, Walder J, Crawford S, Fouayzi H, Mazor KM. Attitudes Toward a Potential SARS-CoV-2 Vaccine. Ann Intern Med 2020; 173(12): 964-73. [http://dx.doi.org/10.7326/M20-3569] [PMID: 32886525]

[33] Malik AA, McFadden SM, Elharake J, Omer SB. Determinants of COVID-19 vaccine acceptance in the US. EClinicalMedicine 2020; 26: 100495. [http://dx.doi.org/10.1016/j.eclinm.2020.100495] [PMID: 32838242]

CHAPTER 6

Computational Drug Discovery Against COVID-19

Shristi Modanwal[1], Viswajit Mulpuru[1] and Nidhi Mishra[1,*]

[1] *Department of Applied Sciences, Indian Institute of Information Technology Allahabad, Prayagraj, India*

Abstract: The global spread of Severe Acute Respiratory Syndrome coronavirus 2 (SARS-CoV-2), which causes the disease COVID-19, has increased drastically since the first cases in Wuhan, People's Republic of China, at the end of 2019. There is no single drug that can be used specifically to treat COVID. The crucial stage in the drug development process is screening huge libraries of bioactive molecules against a biological target, usually a receptor or a protein. Virtual Screening (VS) has become a valuable tool in the drug development process as it allows for efficient *in silico* searches of millions of compounds, resulting in higher yields of possible therapeutic leads, and is cost-effective. The spread of the SARS-CoV-2 virus presents a major threat to world health and has resulted in a global crisis because of the high mortality rate and absence of clinically authorised treatments and vaccines for COVID-19. Finding effective drugs or repurposing available antiviral drugs is a critical need in the fight against COVID-19. VS can be classified as either Structural-Based Virtual Screening or Ligand-Based Virtual Screening. VS techniques have been widely applied in the field of antiviral drug design and have aided in the identification of new compounds as possible anti-viral drugs. Both LBVS and SBVS approaches have proved extremely helpful in identifying several prospective anti-viral drugs with nanomolar range. VS, in contrast to experimental approaches, is quick and cost-effective on the one side but has low prediction accuracy on the other.

Keywords: Ligand-Based Virtual Screening, SARS-CoV-2, Structure-Based Virtual Screening.

INTRODUCTION

Novel drug development is a costly and time-consuming process that can cost billions of dollars and take up to ten years. While most of the money was spent on experimental research to find new drug candidates in the hopes of finding one with biological activity against a target protein a few decades ago, computer-aided drug discovery (CADD) methodologies have garnered interest in recent years because they can reduce the number of ligands that must be tested in experimental

* **Corresponding author Nidhi Mishra:** Indian Institute of Information Technology, Prayagraj, India;
E-mail: nidhimishra@iiita.ac.in

Tahmeena Khan & Alfred J. Lawrence (Eds.)

assays. One of the most essential and extensively used CADD techniques in virtual screening (VS) [1]. VS is an *in-silico* approach for estimating the activity of active molecules/ compounds to identify them. Due to its ability to minimize the cost of screening while also increasing the hit rate, it has become a popular complementary and alternative method to experimental high-throughput screening technologies for drug discovery and development in recent years [2]. Virtual screening uses a large library of small compounds to perform a docking algorithm/calculation to find the conformation and molecular orientation that produces the best score between each small molecule and a target protein. The results are then sorted to provide a list of compounds that are anticipated to bind to a protein target with decreasing strength. To find and validate new drug leads, these predictions can be put to the test in the lab [3]. It also aids in the testing of currently available small compounds for other different diseases. In the field of drug development, VS is one of the most reliable and accurate methods.

A deadly and highly infectious viral disease has recently emerged in Wuhan, China, with the causative agent being identified as a new coronavirus, called Coronavirus disease 2019 (COVID-19) [4, 5]. Resultant of the pandemic of COVID-19, several researchers used a virtual screening approach for drug design and repurposing of pre-existing pharmaceuticals and natural products. The epidemic was so severe that the World Health Organization (WHO) was constrained to designate it as a pandemic just a month after it began to spread widely [6]. The SARS-CoV-2 virus belongs to the order Nidovirales and the family Coronaviridae with a single-stranded positive-sense RNA genome enclosed within a membrane envelope. SARS-CoV-2 is a member of the β coronavirus genus, which also includes the SARS coronavirus (SARS-CoV) and the Middle East respiratory syndrome coronavirus (MERS-CoV) (MERS-CoV) [7]. There are seven types of coronavirus that have been identified as infecting humans (COVID-19) and these are severe acute respiratory syndrome coronavirus (SARS-CoV), Human Coronavirus 229E (HCoV-229E), Human Coronavirus NL63 (HCoV-NL63), Middle East respiratory syndrome coronavirus (MERS-CoV), Human Coronavirus OC43 (HCoV-OC43), Coronavirus Disease 2019 (COVID-19), and Human Coronavirus HKU1 (HCoV-HKU1). Among these, SARS-CoV and MERS-CoV viruses are highly transmissible and pathogenic infections in humans [8]. Coronaviruses cause respiratory, neurological, gastrointestinal systems, and hepatic disorders, as well as serious and sometimes fatal infections. Human-to-human aerosol transmission, which occurs mostly through contaminated droplets, hands, or surfaces, is without a doubt the most common cause of infection. SARS-CoV-2 (novel coronavirus) spreads mostly through the respiratory system and uses Angiotensin-Converting Enzyme 2 (ACE2) receptor, which is the same as SARS-CoV [9].

Consequently, the number of affected people continues to rise, and no effective treatments have yet been discovered. As a result, the need for medications to treat COVID-19 is critical. The coronavirus has the most significant structural proteins, namely Spike Proteins(S), Membrane Proteins (M), NucleocapsidProteins (N), and Envelope Proteins (E) [10]. These proteins are required for viral genome replication, synthesis, virion, and viroporin formation, virion-receptor attachment, which all contribute to the virus's ability to enter and multiply in a host organism, spreading infection [11]. In addition to mentioned structural proteins, replicase proteins, Main protease or Chymotrypsin-like protease (Mpro or 3CLpro), and papain-like protease (PLPRO) play an important role in the pathogenesis of SARS-CoV-2 [12]. Proteins such as Rna-directed RNA polymerase (RdRp) and Non-structural protein 15 (nsp15), nsp 16 can also be used as targets. SARS HCoV has the RdRp that is most similar to SARS-CoV-2, so the SARS-Co--2RdRp model should be built as a homolog of the SARS HCoVRdRp [13].

VIRTUAL SCREENING METHODS

Virtual screening is currently a standard procedure in drug discovery before wet-lab studies. When several drug candidates, and other drug-like small molecules bind to a specific protein, Virtual Screening is used to short-list significant candidates by estimating the estimated affinities and possible binding mechanisms of these compounds. Even while VS is far less expensive than lab research, it still necessitates the installation of appropriate High-Performance Computing infrastructure to screen huge ligand libraries [14]. The availability of high-resolution structures of many of the SARS-CoV-2 proteins aided us in quickly identifying lead therapeutic candidates for SARS-CoV-2 using *in silico* screening methods. Virtual Screening can be Structural Based Virtual Screening (SBVS) and Ligand Based Virtual Screening (LBVS). Based on structural activity data from a pool of known active compounds, LBVS identifies promising compounds for laboratory experiments. The LBVS method includes quantitative structure-activity relationship (QSAR), pharmacophore mapping, similarity and substructure searches, and 3D shape matching. SBVS, on the other hand, docks potential molecules and ranks them according to their expected binding affinity to the binding site utilizing the biological target's 3D structure, which was either determined experimentally through X-ray crystallography or NMR or computationally through homology modeling [15, 16]. SBVS is the best approach for discovering novel ligands when the target protein's 3D structure has been experimentally determined. When the target's 3D structure is unknown or prediction using structure-based approaches is problematic, LBVS is the best procedure [1]. A schematic representation of Virtual Screening and its categories is shown in (Fig. **1**).

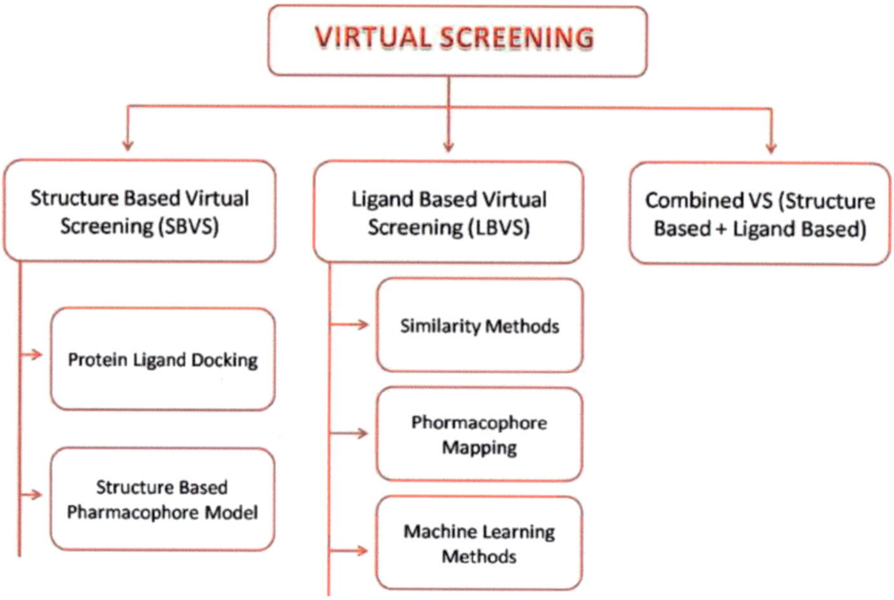

Fig. (1). Schematic representation of virtual screening.

Structure-Based Virtual Screening

SBVS begins by analyzing the 3D target structural data of interest. Experimental data could be used to derive the target structure. When considering a biological target for SBVS, many fundamental issues should be considered, including the receptor's drug ability, binding site selection, protein structure selection, incorporating receptor flexibility, appropriate protonation state assignment, and consideration of water molecules in a binding site [17]. SBVS can be further mainly divided into two categories, including Protein-Ligand Docking and Structure-Based Pharmacophore.

Protein-Ligand Docking

Protein-Ligand Docking, also referred to as molecular docking, is a widely popular approach in the drug discovery field because it can process vast compound libraries in a reasonable amount of time. DOCK, GOLD, Glide, AutoDock Vina, Maestro Schrodinger, FlexX, ICM, LigandFit, Glide, Surflex, rDock, and eHiTS are some of the most popular docking programs. The primary inputs of typical docking are a target protein structure that has been experimentally determined or computationally modelled and a small molecule compound library that can be synthesized or purchased. Considering drug development against COVID-19, the desired proteins should include Spike Proteins, Membrane Proteins, Nucleocapsid Proteins, Envelope Proteins,

Replicase proteins, Main protease or Chymotrypsin-like protease (Mpro or 3CLpro), Papain-like Protease (PLPRO), Rna-directed RNA polymerase (RdRp) and Non-structural protein 15 (nsp15), nsp16. The targets can be downloaded from the protein data bank in PDB format and the ligands/compounds can be downloaded from PubChem, ZINC databank, *etc*, in SDF format. Before performing docking, targets, as well as compounds, should be prepared; this includes assigning proper tautomeric, stereoisomeric, and protonation states. Each molecule is virtually docked into the protein's active site using docking software that models the protein-ligand interactions to achieve optimal steric and physicochemical compatibility. This is frequently followed by a post-processing process in which compounds are evaluated and selected based on calculated binding scores and/or other criteria. The top-ranked compounds are being picked as potent candidates for subsequent experimental studies [18]. Docking programs estimate the location, orientation, and internal conformation of small molecules in a protein's binding site. The protein is rigid or semi-rigid, enabling certain selected groups to rotate to improve hydrogen bonding. A search algorithm like Genetic Algorithm or Monte Carlo search is used by docking software to examine alternative ligand postures for the binding site, which are subsequently scored using a scoring function to measure the force of non-covalent interactions between protein and ligand. The scoring function includes force-field-based, knowledge-based, and empirical criteria (scoring) [19, 20]. Further, the lead compound identified through docking analysis can be subjected to Molecular Dynamic Simulation for stability validation. The graphical representation of docking is given in (Fig. **2**).

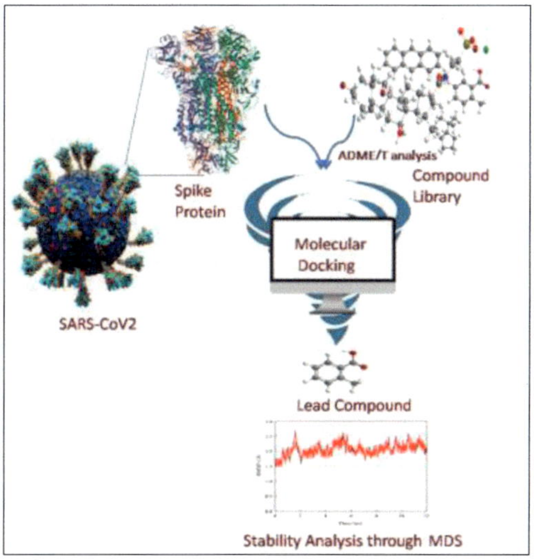

Fig. (2). Screening of large compound library to get lead compound through Protein-Ligand Docking.

Structure-Based Pharmacophores

The 3D structure of a protein, when interacting with its docked ligand, is typically used in structure-based pharmacophore modelling. As a result, the pharmacophore can incorporate more comprehensive information about the ligand's accessible areas. Pharmit is an online server that virtually screens numerous drug databases utilizing pharmacophore models, molecular morphologies, and energy minimization [21]. Structure-based pharmacophore modelling combines the benefits of both ligand and structure-based methods [22]. Some methods can be used to obtain the properties that will construct the Structure-Based Pharmacophore, like using the amino acid residues in binding sites of the protein; it includes the receptor, not the ligands, which provides the pharmacophore characteristics. This approach allows pharmacophores obtained from distinct crystallographic structures of the same target to be compared. Another is by using co-crystallized ligand conformations with receptors; the pharmacophore properties are also derived from active molecules, but because they are co-crystallized with the receptor, their bioactive conformations are already known and no conformations need to be generated. The pharmacophore properties also can be generated by docking fragments into the receptor's binding site; it uses a cluster of docked fragments [23]. Rampogu S *et al.* [24] built a structure-based pharmacophore model by taking advantage of interacting properties between nsp16/nsp10 complexed and co-crystallized ligand SAM. As a result of the findings, ten pharmacophore models with similar characteristics have been generated. A total of 37 characteristics in ligands were discovered when the receptor-ligand complex generation protocol was started. Six of the ten properties that matched the receptor-ligand interactions were integrated into each model: AAAAAADDPP (A is hydrogen bond acceptor, D is hydrogen bond donor, and P represents positively ionizable). The rules, an internal scoring technique, were employed as the scoring method. The pharmacophore that covered the whole structure of the SAM, as well as the crucial residue interactions, was selected to be the best model. The ligand's properties were compatible with the target's critical residues. The model's ability to find potential inhibitors was then tested. The pan-MTase inhibitor sinefungin was employed because there are few drugs specific to the nsp16/nsp10 complex. The nsp10-nsp16methyl transferase complex of SARS-CoV-2 binds this molecule.

Ligand-Based Virtual Screening

The LBVS approach is predicated on the concept of small-molecule similarity. Similar ligands have similar biological properties. This model can then be used to identify new ligands with similar properties. When we only have a small number of known ligands, these approaches work poorly [25]. It uses structure-activity data from a set of known active molecules to identify likely drug candidates for experimental confirmation. Similarity method, pharmacophore mapping, machine learning method are some of the strategies that have been utilized in the LBSV method [26].

Similarity Method

In the drug development trade, similarity methods are widely used to identify suitable drug candidates since it is assumed that molecules with identical structural characteristics will have similar properties. Similarity methods are used for drug repurposing. Molecular similarity analysis typically requires the definition of descriptors that represent molecules, as well as a method for measuring the level of similarity between molecules. Depending on the molecular representations used to calculate them, many types of descriptors have been developed, which can be classified as one-dimensional (1D), two-dimensional (2D), three-dimensional (3D), and four-dimensional (4D). 1D descriptors include basic molecular properties like molecular weight, size, BCUT parameters, dipole moment, and so on. While others, such as 2D descriptors, simplify atomic information in them. The molecular volume and surface properties can be simplified by 3D descriptors and 3D coordinates and conformations can be simplified by 4D descriptors [27, 28]. Dragon, CDK toolkit, PaDEL, and RDKit are some software for descriptors. The two widely used similarity methods in ligand-based virtual screening are 2D fingerprints and 3D shape. The binary fragment information on a known ligand is used in 2D fingerprint-based virtual screening.

Although the COVID-19 vaccine is still being rolled out over the world, there is still a need to find effective therapies, especially in areas where vaccination uptake is poor and where the threat of vaccine escape from mutations is present. As the pandemic's urgency makes the development of novel medications nearly impossible, repurposing existing drugs to treat COVID-19 is an appealing method, particularly if they are already authorized and have a well range of safety. The basic procedure of *in silico* drug repurposing is shown in (Fig. **3**). There are many research articles in which the similarity methods were applied to repurpose the existing drug to predict the drug for COVID-19 [29 - 31]. Meng Y *et al.* [32] use SMILES (Simplified Molecular Input Line Entry System) for similarity purposes. SMILES describe the molecular structure of a compound. The chemical structure information of drugs has been downloaded from the DrugBank database in SMILE format. The Molecular Access System (MACCS) fingerprints of each drug were then calculated using Open Babel v2.3.1. The similarity between the two compounds was measured by using the Tanimoto index.

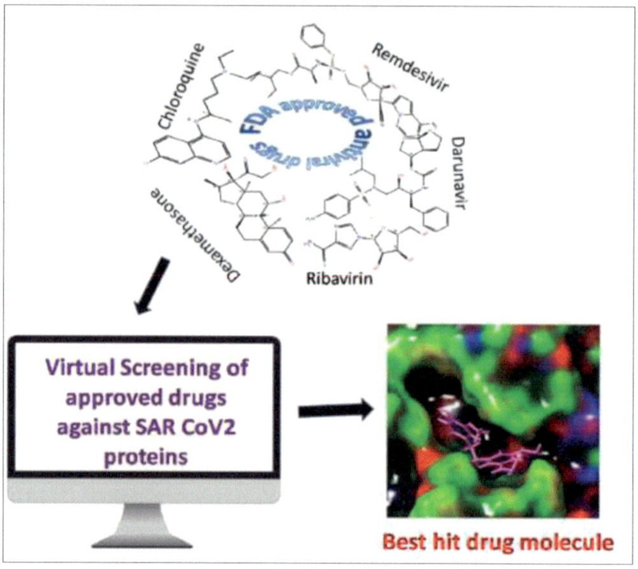

Fig. (3). Basic representation of *in silico* drug repurposing.

Pharmacophore Mapping

The spatial arrangement of the elemental composition of ligands that are essential for interaction with the target receptor is shown by a pharmacophore model. Hydrophobic regions, Hydrogen bond donors, hydrogen bond acceptors, positively charged ionizable groups, negatively charged ionizable groups, and aromatic ring systems are some of the chemical properties employed in pharmacophore modelling. The pharmacophore model might include the bioactive conformation of the molecules within the target binding site. Catalyst, PHASE, LigandScout, GALAHAD, PHASE, ZINC Pharmer, and PharmMapper are some of the most often used software for building pharmacophore models automatically. A good pharmacophore model also includes spatial limitations in regions inhabited by inactive molecules, which are frequently improved to make the model less restrictive. All pharmacophoric properties that aren't consistently found inactive compounds are either left out of the final model or made optional [33]. Pharmacophores can be used in a variety of ways in drug development programs, including (1) a 3D query tool in virtual screening to find potential new lead compounds from 3D databases of "drug-like" molecules with a patentable configuration that are different from those already discovered; (2) to predict the activities of a group of new compounds that have yet to be synthesized; (3) to analyze the possible mode of action [34]. Pharmacophore modelling has been used in COVID-19 drug prediction process. Haider Z *et al.* [35] built a pharmacophore model by ZINC pharmacophore to screen best-hit compounds with a similar feature of the reference combination of receptor Mpro with N3 inhibitor from the ZINC database. To build a pharmacophore model, the main properties of one hydrophobic, one H-accepter, one H-donor, and one aromatic were chosen, and the ZINC database, which contains over 250 million chemicals in 3D format, was screened. 1500 hit compounds were found, and then Lipinski's thumb rule of five resulted in the selection of 700 out of 1500 hit compounds. The energy minimization algorithm in MOE using force-field MMFF94x, with Gradient 0.05, was used to shift all hits into a test database.

Machine Learning Method

The use of various machine learning algorithms in drug discovery has benefited pharmaceutical companies greatly. In the field of drug development, machine learning (ML) has been utilized to construct numerous models for predicting the biological, chemical, and physical properties of compounds. ML can be used in all stages of the drug development process, including finding novel uses for pharmaceuticals, predicting drug-protein interactions, discovering drug efficacy, ensuring safety biomarkers, and optimizing molecular bioactivity. Random Forest (RF), Naive Bayesian (NB), QSAR ML, and support vector machine (SVM) are examples of machine learning techniques that have been frequently employed in drug development [36]. Several FDA-approved drugs have been screened computationally for SARS-CoV-2 treatment. Sovesh M *et al.* [37] applied the ML approach for repurposing FDA-approved drugs as a test model to predict new drugs for COVID 19. They used inhibitors of the SARS Coronavirus 3C-like Protease to train their model. Naive Bayes algorithm was used for training and prediction of FDA-approved drugs and identified Amprenavir as a possible candidate for limiting viral identification of host cells or disrupting host-virus interactions. There are recent studies where machine learning techniques are used to predict pharmacokinetic activity [38]. In this study, a large and diverse dataset of drug compounds is used to model a prediction model of fraction unbound drugs in plasma using chemical fingerprints. Building machine learning models using the quantitative structure-activity relationship (QSAR) method on promising protein targets of the SARS-CoV-2 virus could predict potential therapeutic candidates for COVID-19 treatment. In LBVS, the Quantitative structure-activity relationships (QSAR) study is the most effective approach because of its high and fast throughput as well as a high hit rate. Essential chemogenomics data is gathered from databases and the research/literature as the first preliminary stage in the building of a QSAR model. Then chemical descriptors were derived on several levels of molecular structure representation, ranging from 1D to nD, and associated with the biological feature [39].

Combined LBVS and SBVS

The Structure and Ligand Based Virtual Screening can be combined to make the virtual screening more powerful. The combined VS can be carried out since both the ligand and the target structure are available. There are so many works that have been published for COVID 19 drug development by the combined method. Onat Kadioglu *et al.* [40] selected the target proteins of SARS-CoV-2 and built a homology model of the protein. Constructed a drug library of FDA-approved drugs, as well as natural products, taken from ZINC database and literature, respectively, a total of 41134 compounds have been taken. The selected compounds were subjected to Molecular docking using PyRx AutoDock VINA to study the interaction between protein and ligand. Top 100 compounds were taken to check drug-likeness property using supervised machine learning. The well-scored compounds have been identified as candidate compounds against SARS-CoV-2.

INTERPRETING DRUG INTERACTION

A molecular docking study can be performed to examine the interaction between a protein and a ligand. It also shows the types of interactions, as well as interacting residues and atoms. The interactions can be hydrophobic, hydrogen bonding, pi-pi stacking, *etc*. We studied the COVID-19 main protease inhibitors found in Tinospora cordifolia, considering Remdesivir and Favipiravir as control, which are promising medications that have been shown to inhibit COVID-19. The interaction diagram which has been shown (Fig. **4**) is from our study [41]. The interaction diagram shows that remdesivir interacts with HIS 164, GLY 143, ARG 188, MET 135, *etc*., and also forms a hydrogen bond with GLN 189, THR 24, and THR 26 amino acid residues of COVID-19 main protease.

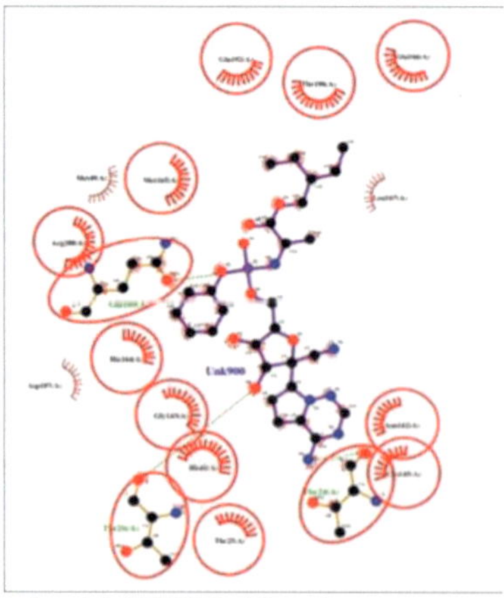

Fig. (4). Interaction of Remdesivir with COVID-19 main protease.

APPLICATION OF VIRTUAL SCREENING FOR COVID 19 THERAPEUTICS

- Akhilesh *et al.* – the authors have screened various coumarin derivatives against different SARS-CoV-2 proteins such as Main Protease, NSP10/ NSP16-Methyltransferase, Phosphatase, and Endoribonuclease to identify their inhibitors [42].
- Viswajit *et al.*- In this study, the phytochemicals from a few medicinal plants in India have been screened against the main protease of SARS-CoV-2 to identify potential inhibitors [41].
- Santosh *et al.*- This study screens a few anti-viral, anti-infectious, and anti-protease compounds for repurposing against NSP10/NSP16 methyltransferase and main protease of SARS-CoV 2 [43].
- Iqbal Azad *et al.*- this study sets out to identify potential inhibitors from natural food sources against the main protease of SARS-CoV-2, SARS-CoV, MERS-CoV, and HCoV-HKV1 [44].
- Viswajit *et al.*- the authors have identified potential vaccine epitope candidates from the Indian isolates of SARS-CoV-2 and further validated the immunogenicity of the epitope candidates for vaccine development [45].
- Md. Mahbubur Rahman *et al.*- In this study, the authors have set to repurpose the FDA-approved drugs against the main protease of SARS-CoV-2. Further, the authors constructed a predictive QSAR model [46].

FUTURE PROSPECTS OF VIRTUAL SCREENING

Considering the numerous steps of VS detailed in this study, it is evident that the entire process is dependent on a mix of various types of analysis, data, and filters. We will be able to process large quantities of virtual compounds quickly using the capacity to combine several filters. VS techniques frequently required meticulous training set preparation, careful parameter selection, and proper analysis of the outcomes. It is impossible for someone who does not have a thorough understanding of the software's internal workings and underlying theory to utilise it successfully and provide meaningful results. This development has the potential as a future technology to help medical experts in the selection of the most effective drugs or to help those with fewer side effects for individual patients. It has wide applications in many fields, such as transgenic animal studies, cancer tissue microarrays and other diseases, and normal tissues and cells during development. This approach can be used to develop new and potent drugs.

CONCLUSION

With the advancements in computers, virtual screening has become a valuable tool in drug discovery. Known for its efficiency, virtual screening techniques are known to provide economical and time-efficient methods for the discovery of novel compounds. Particularly, because of the cost and time required for drug development, virtual screening methods are extensively being incorporated in the drug-discovery studies. The recent advances in the computational power required for ligand conformation searching, receptor flexibility analysis, and cheminformatics data analysis continue has prioritized the virtual screening techniques in drug design & discovery.

With SARS-CoV-2 infections leading to about 50,00,000 deaths worldwide in over 200 countries, Virtual screening is a highly efficient tool to identify potential antiviral compounds. Therefore, the use of these techniques is necessary to find and evaluate treatment methods quickly. The binding predictions and the ranking of drugs will be useful in the interpretation of the results to accelerate the time required for clinical trials. In conclusion, virtual screening techniques such as molecular docking, molecular dynamics simulation, and the ADME / pharmacokinetic analysis would lead to the identification of drugs for general treatments and coronavirus-specific treatments along with other antiviral treatments rapidly with cost-effectiveness.

CONSENT FOR PUBLICATION

Not applicable.

CONFLICT OF INTEREST

The authors declare no conflict of interest, financial or otherwise.

ACKNOWLEDGEMENT

Uttar Pradesh Council of Science and Technology.

REFERENCES

[1] Banegas-Luna AJ, Cerón-Carrasco JP, Pérez-Sánchez H. A review of ligand-based virtual screening web tools and screening algorithms in large molecular databases in the age of big data. Future Med Chem 2018; 10(22): 2641-58. [http://dx.doi.org/10.4155/fmc-2018-0076] [PMID: 30499744]

[2] Li J, Liu W, Song Y, Xia J. Improved method of structure-based virtual screening based on ensemble learning. RSC Advances 2020; 10(13): 7609-18. [http://dx.doi.org/10.1039/C9RA09211K] [PMID: 35492172]

[3] Viswanathan U, Tomlinson SM, Fonner JM, Mock SA, Watowich SJ. Identification of a novel inhibitor of dengue virus protease through use of a virtual screening drug discovery Web portal. J Chem Inf Model 2014; 54(10): 2816-25. [http://dx.doi.org/10.1021/ci500531r] [PMID: 25263519]

[4] Kandeel M, Al-Nazawi M. Virtual screening and repurposing of FDA approved drugs against COVID-19 main protease. Life Sci 2020; 251: 117627.

[http://dx.doi.org/10.1016/j.lfs.2020.117627] [PMID: 32251634]

[5] Zhang S, Li L, Shen A, Chen Y, Qi Z. Rational Use of Tocilizumab in the Treatment of Novel Coronavirus Pneumonia. Clin Drug Investig 2020; 40(6): 511-8. [http://dx.doi.org/10.1007/s40261-020-00917-3] [PMID: 32337664]

[6] Nguyen DC, Ding M, Pathirana PN, *et al.* Federated Learning for Industrial Internet of Things in Future Industries. IEEE Wirel Commun 2021; 28(6): 192-9. [http://dx.doi.org/10.1109/MWC.001.2100102]

[7] Pal M, Berhanu G, Desalegn C, Kandi V. Severe Acute Respiratory Syndrome Coronavirus-2 (SARS-CoV-2): An Update. Cureus 2020; 12(3): e7423. [http://dx.doi.org/10.7759/cureus.7423] [PMID: 32337143]

[8] Mao X, Guo L, Fu P, Xiang C. The status and trends of coronavirus research. Medicine (Baltimore) 2020; 99(22): e20137. [http://dx.doi.org/10.1097/MD.0000000000020137] [PMID: 32481379]

[9] Marinho EM, Batista de Andrade Neto J, Silva J, *et al.* Virtual screening based on molecular docking of possible inhibitors of Covid-19 main protease. Microb Pathog 2020; 148: 104365. [http://dx.doi.org/10.1016/j.micpath.2020.104365] [PMID: 32619669]

[10] Mariano G, Farthing RJ, Lale-Farjat SLM, Bergeron JRC. Structural Characterization of SARS-Co--2: Where We Are, and Where We Need to Be. Front Mol Biosci 2020; 7: 605236. [http://dx.doi.org/10.3389/fmolb.2020.605236] [PMID: 33392262]

[11] Satarker S, Nampoothiri M. Structural Proteins in Severe Acute Respiratory Syndrome Coronavirus-2. Arch Med Res 2020; 51(6): 482-91. [http://dx.doi.org/10.1016/j.arcmed.2020.05.012] [PMID: 32493627]

[12] Shamsi A, Mohammad T, Anwar S, *et al.* Potential drug targets of SARS-CoV-2: From genomics to therapeutics. Int J Biol Macromol 2021; 177: 1-9. [http://dx.doi.org/10.1016/j.ijbiomac.2021.02.071] [PMID: 33577820]

[13] Quimque MTJ, Notarte KIR, Fernandez RAT, *et al.* Virtual screening-driven drug discovery of SARS-CoV-2 enzyme inhibitors targeting viral attachment, replication, post-translational modification and host immunity evasion infection mechanisms. J Biomol Struct Dyn 2021; 39(12): 4316-33. [http://dx.doi.org/10.1080/07391102.2020.1776639] [PMID: 32476574]

[14] Jaghoori MM, Bleijlevens B, Olabarriaga SD. 1001 Ways to run AutoDock Vina for virtual screening. J Comput Aided Mol Des 2016; 30(3): 237-49. [http://dx.doi.org/10.1007/s10822-016-9900-9] [PMID: 26897747]

[15] Trabocchi A, Ed. Small molecule drug discovery. Waltham: Elsevier 2019.

[16] Scior T, Bender A, Tresadern G, *et al.* Recognizing pitfalls in virtual screening: a critical review. J Chem Inf Model 2012; 52(4): 867-81. [http://dx.doi.org/10.1021/ci200528d] [PMID: 22435959]

[17] Lionta E, Spyrou G, Vassilatis D, Cournia Z. Structure-based virtual screening for drug discovery: principles, applications and recent advances. Curr Top Med Chem 2014; 14(16): 1923-38. [http://dx.doi.org/10.2174/1568026614666140929124445] [PMID: 25262799]

[18] Cheng T, Li Q, Zhou Z, Wang Y, Bryant SH. Structure-based virtual screening for drug discovery: a problem-centric review. AAPS J 2012; 14(1): 133-41. [http://dx.doi.org/10.1208/s12248-012-9322-0] [PMID: 22281989]

[19] Varela-Rial A, Majewski M, De Fabritiis G. Structure based virtual screening: Fast and slow. Wiley Interdiscip Rev Comput Mol Sci 2021. [http://dx.doi.org/10.1002/wcms.1544]

[20] Wu CH, Arighi CN, Ross KE, Eds. Protein bioinformatics: from protein modifications and networks to proteomics. New York: Humana Press 2017.

[http://dx.doi.org/10.1007/978-1-4939-6783-4]

[21] Shiri F, Pirhadi S, Ghasemi JB. Dynamic structure based pharmacophore modeling of the Acetylcholinesterase reveals several potential inhibitors. J Biomol Struct Dyn 2019; 37(7): 1800-12. [http://dx.doi.org/10.1080/07391102.2018.1468281] [PMID: 29695192]

[22] Kayık G, Tüzün NŞ, Durdagi S. Investigation of PDE5/PDE6 and PDE5/PDE11 selective potent tadalafil-like PDE5 inhibitors using combination of molecular modeling approaches, molecular fingerprint-based virtual screening protocols and structure-based pharmacophore development. J Enzyme Inhib Med Chem 2017; 32(1): 311-30. [http://dx.doi.org/10.1080/14756366.2016.1250756] [PMID: 28150511]

[23] Gimeno A, Ojeda-Montes M, Tomás-Hernández S, *et al.* The Light and Dark Sides of Virtual Screening: What Is There to Know? Int J Mol Sci 2019; 20(6): 1375. [http://dx.doi.org/10.3390/ijms20061375] [PMID: 30893780]

[24] Rampogu S, Lee KW. Pharmacophore Modelling-Based Drug Repurposing Approaches for SARS-CoV-2 Therapeutics. Front Chem 2021; 9: 636362. [http://dx.doi.org/10.3389/fchem.2021.636362] [PMID: 34041221]

[25] Grinter S, Zou X. Challenges, applications, and recent advances of protein-ligand docking in structure-based drug design. Molecules 2014; 19(7): 10150-76. [http://dx.doi.org/10.3390/molecules190710150] [PMID: 25019558]

[26] Khan AU. Virtual Screening Strategies: A State of Art to Combat with Multiple Drug Resistance Strains. MOJPB 2015; 2: pp. (2)61-6. [http://dx.doi.org/10.15406/mojpb.2015.02.00042]

[27] Garcia-Hernandez C, Fernández A, Serratosa F. Ligand-Based Virtual Screening Using Graph Edit Distance as Molecular Similarity Measure. J Chem Inf Model 2019; 59(4): 1410-21. [http://dx.doi.org/10.1021/acs.jcim.8b00820] [PMID: 30920214]

[28] Hussin SK, Omar YM, Abdelmageid SM, Marie MI. Traditional machine learning and big data analytics in virtual screening: a comparative study. Int J Adv Comput Res 2020; 10(47): 72-88. [http://dx.doi.org/10.19101/IJACR.2019.940150]

[29] Meyer-Almes FJ. Repurposing approved drugs as potential inhibitors of 3CL-protease of SARS-Co--2: Virtual screening and structure based drug design. Comput Biol Chem 2020; 88: 107351. [http://dx.doi.org/10.1016/j.compbiolchem.2020.107351] [PMID: 32769050]

[30] Jang WD, Jeon S, Kim S, Lee SY. Drugs repurposed for COVID-19 by virtual screening of 6,218 drugs and cell-based assay. Proc Natl Acad Sci USA 2021; 118(30): e2024302118. [http://dx.doi.org/10.1073/pnas.2024302118] [PMID: 34234012]

[31] Wang Y, Sun Y, Wang Y, Ju Y, Meng D. Virtual screening of active compounds from Artemisia argyi and potential targets against gastric ulcer based on Network pharmacology. Bioorg Chem 2019; 88: 102924. [http://dx.doi.org/10.1016/j.bioorg.2019.102924] [PMID: 31005783]

[32] Meng Y, Jin M, Tang X, Xu J. Drug repositioning based on similarity constrained probabilistic matrix factorization: COVID-19 as a case study. Appl Soft Comput 2021; 103: 107135. [http://dx.doi.org/10.1016/j.asoc.2021.107135] [PMID: 33519322]

[33] Gurung AB, Ali MA, Lee J, Farah MA, Al-Anazi KM. An Updated Review of Computer-Aided Drug Design and Its Application to COVID-19. BioMed Res Int 2021; 2021: 1-18. [http://dx.doi.org/10.1155/2021/8853056] [PMID: 34258282]

[34] Yadav D, Paliwal S, Yadav R, Pal M, Pandey A. Identification of novel HIV 1--protease inhibitors: application of ligand and structure based pharmacophore mapping and virtual screening. PLoS One 2012; 7(11): e48942. [http://dx.doi.org/10.1371/journal.pone.0048942] [PMID: 23145032]

[35] Haider Z, Subhani MM, Farooq MA, Ishaq M, Khalid M, Khan RSA, *et al. In Silico* Discovery of

Novel Inhibitors Against Main Protease (M^{pro}) of SARS-CoV-2 Using Pharmacophore and Molecular Docking Based Virtual Screening from zinc database. Medicine & Pharmacology 2020. [http://dx.doi.org/10.20944/preprints202002.0431.v1]

[36] Patel L, Shukla T, Huang X, Ussery DW, Wang S. Machine Learning Methods in Drug Discovery. Molecules 2020; 25(22): 5277. [http://dx.doi.org/10.3390/molecules25225277] [PMID: 33198233]

[37] Mohapatra S, Nath P, Chatterjee M, *et al.* Repurposing therapeutics for COVID-19: Rapid prediction of commercially available drugs through machine learning and docking. PLoS One 2020; 15(11): e0241543. [http://dx.doi.org/10.1371/journal.pone.0241543] [PMID: 33180803]

[38] Mulpuru V, Mishra N. *In Silico* Prediction of Fraction Unbound in Human Plasma from Chemical Fingerprint Using Automated Machine Learning. ACS Omega 2021; 6(10): 6791-7. [http://dx.doi.org/10.1021/acsomega.0c05846] [PMID: 33748592]

[39] Neves BJ, Braga RC, Melo-Filho CC, Moreira-Filho JT, Muratov EN, Andrade CH. QSAR-Based Virtual Screening: Advances and Applications in Drug Discovery. Front Pharmacol 2018; 9: 1275. [http://dx.doi.org/10.3389/fphar.2018.01275] [PMID: 30524275]

[40] Kadioglu O, Saeed M, Greten HJ, Efferth T. Identification of novel compounds against three targets of SARS CoV-2 coronavirus by combined virtual screening and supervised machine learning. Comput Biol Med 2021; 133: 104359. [http://dx.doi.org/10.1016/j.compbiomed.2021.104359] [PMID: 33845270]

[41] Mulpuru V, Mishra N. Computational Identification of SARS-CoV-2 Inhibitor in *Tinospora cordifolia, Cinnamomum zeylanicum and Myristica fragrans.* Virusdisease 2021; 32(3): 511-7. [http://dx.doi.org/10.1007/s13337-021-00721-3] [PMID: 34337109]

[42] Maurya AK, Mishra N. *In silico* validation of coumarin derivatives as potential inhibitors against Main Protease, NSP10/NSP16-Methyltransferase, Phosphatase and Endoribonuclease of SARS CoV-2. J Biomol Struct Dyn 2020; 1-16. [http://dx.doi.org/10.1080/07391102.2020.1808075] [PMID: 32835632]

[43] Maurya SK, Maurya AK, Mishra N, Siddique HR. Virtual screening, ADME/T, and binding free energy analysis of anti-viral, anti-protease, and anti-infectious compounds against NSP10/NSP16 methyltransferase and main protease of SARS CoV-2. J Recept Signal Transduct Res 2020; 40(6): 605-12. [http://dx.doi.org/10.1080/10799893.2020.1772298] [PMID: 32476594]

[44] Azad I, Khan T, Maurya AK, Irfan Azad M, Mishra N, Alanazi AM. Identification of Severe Acute Respiratory Syndrome Coronavirus-2 inhibitors through *in silico* structure-based virtual screening and molecular interaction studies. J Mol Recognit 2021; 34(10): e2918. [http://dx.doi.org/10.1002/jmr.2918] [PMID: 34132436]

[45] Mulpuru V, Mishra N. Immunoinformatic based identification of cytotoxic T lymphocyte epitopes from the Indian isolate of SARS-CoV-2. Sci Rep 2021; 11(1): 4516. [http://dx.doi.org/10.1038/s41598-021-83949-9] [PMID: 33633155]

[46] Rahman MM, Saha T, Islam KJ, *et al.* Virtual screening, molecular dynamics and structure–activity relationship studies to identify potent approved drugs for Covid-19 treatment. J Biomol Struct Dyn 2021; 39(16): 6231-41. [http://dx.doi.org/10.1080/07391102.2020.1794974] [PMID: 32692306]

CHAPTER 7

Methods in Drug Repurposing: Emphasis on COVID-19

Akhilesh Kumar Maurya[1] and **Nidhi Mishra**[1,*]

[1] *Chemistry Laboratory, Department of Applied Sciences, Indian Institute of Information Technology Allahabad, Prayagraj, 211012, India*

Abstract: Coronavirus disease 19 (COVID-19) is a pandemic situation caused by the SARS-CoV-2 (severe acute respiratory syndrome coronavirus 2), and dedicated medical research finding to cure the disease are rapidly evolving globally. SARS-Co--2 is a highly mutating virus having various strains, till the reporting of this study, COVID-19 has 5 variants, *i.e.*, Alfa, beta, gamma, delta, and omicron. A potential way for drug development is drug repurposing has got a lot of attention. Drug repurposing is the easiest and safest way to find out the drugs to cure COVID-19. Various new drugs have been discovered and are under clinical trial for the treatment of disease. Combinatorial treatments of COVID-19 patients give a very positive response in the treatment of SARS-CoV-2. The various vaccine already has been developed to produce antibodies against COVID-19. However, a large number of research studies have been done on COVID-19. This study is dedicated to research on COVID-19 therapy by the repurposing of existing drugs and methods used for the drug repurposing.

Keywords: Combinatorial, COVID-19, Drug Repurposing, Medical Research, SARS-CoV-2, Targeted Based Approaches.

INTRODUCTION

The pandemic potential of new or mutated viruses has been increasing over the past few decades, as evidenced by epidemic and pandemic storms of the Middle East respiratory virus (MERS-CoV), Human Immunodeficiency Virus (HIV), Ebola virus (EBOV), Zika virus (ZIKV), for which we have still no drugs or lack of specific therapy [1]. World Health Organization (WHO) endeavour to be "the global guardian of health" are repeatedly conquered by the arrival of COVID-19 disease caused by the coronavirus. With over 2.4 Billion confirmed COVID-19 cases and 4.8 million people death recorded worldwide [2] and counting continues, the pandemic outbreak of COVID-19 was declared by WHO on March 11, 2020 [3]. Albeit huge advancements have been made to comprehend

* **Corresponding author Nidhi Mishra:** Chemistry Laboratory, Department of Applied Sciences, Indian Institute of Information Technology Allahabad, Prayagraj, 211012, India; E-mail: nidhimishra@iiita.ac.in

Tahmeena Khan & Alfred J. Lawrence (Eds.)

and cure Coronavirus, the flow pandemic has, generally, overpowered drug organizations to facilitate the improvement of antibodies and medications against this clever sickness. The lethargic speed in clever medication advancement, combined with high steady loss rates and expanding administrative obstacles, has provoked medication engineers to consider another medication improvement technique: drug repurposing.

The COVID-19 virus is a capsulated RNA (ribonucleic acid) virus, from the genus β-coronavirus, *i.e.*, present in bats, aves, and other mammals, including humans [4]. Coronavirus have four subfamilies: δ (delta), ϒ (gamma), β (beta), and α (alpha) coronaviruses. Among these, α and β-coronavirus come from mammals, especially from bats; ϒ and δ- variant of coronaviruses arise from pigs and aves [5]. Coronavirus has a genome of single-stranded RNA (ssRNA) that is confined with a capsulated structure of proteins [6].

Designing and developing new therapeutic drugs with an exhaustive profile of the COVID-19 virus is a time-taking, costly, and challenging process. To reduce these, drug repurposing (also known as repositioning or rediscovery) is an interesting way to accelerate the recognition of drugs from the existing databases of drugs that can cure or treat COVID-19 [7]. Drug repurposing or repositioning may help us to find new therapeutics for any diseases in a short time with low costs, basically when the clinical and or preclinical and trials and safety test experiments have been completed for drug molecules [8]. The basic motto of drug repositioning is to hike the curative use of previously usable medicine for more and new medical treatment purposes [9]. Computational approaches for repurposing drugs attempt new testable expectations for the standardized reuse of available tested drugs [10].

Drug Repurposing Methods

Like every drug repurposing project, Drugs repurposing under COVID-19 follow these three steps [11]:

1. Identifying the candidate drug;
2. Mechanistic evaluation of the preclinical models of effect drug; and
3. Assessment of the drug candidature.

The systematic approach to the re-use of medicines is widely divided into *in silico/* computational and experimental methods. However, it should be recognized that these methods can be utilized in synergy to obtain the foremost reassignment result.

Computational Methods

Structure-Based

Possibly one of the most common approaches to reallocating medications in the pandemic of SARS-CoV-2 disease. Structure-based screening analyses for SARS-CoV-2 inhibitors have been highly recorded in numerous research studies worldwide, due to the high computing capacity and availability of three-dimensional structures of drug molecules and receptor target proteins and nucleic acid [12]. Structure-based screening of ligands or drug molecules is an *in silico* method used in the initial phase of a medication repurposing drive to look for biologically active compounds against certain therapeutic targets, based on receptor binding site complementarity in a compound library. This computational virtual screening can be done in two steps [13].

1. Molecular docking is carried out on many previously available drugs or drug library applicants to link the 3-D structure of a target receptor obtained by NMR, X-ray approaches, or computational modelling methods.
2. A score of binding affinity is used to compute the probability of all drugs/ligands connecting the target molecule with high affinity, giving antique repurposing hits.

Because of knowledge of its antecedents (SARS-CoV-2 and MERS-CoV), the cellular targets are very well defined. This target-centric strategy is particularly useful, potentially eliminating the necessity to illuminate the action mode of hits. As a result, several medications may be tested against a specific target receptor (such as Angiotensin-Converting Enzyme-2 (ACE2), Main Protease), as in the normal docking method. Elfiky used ordinary sub-molecular docking techniques, including coronavirus RNA-dependent RNA polymerase (RdRP), to evaluate for expected drug molecules such as SARS-CoV-2 inhibitors, virtual screening presently supported inhibitors of polymerase medications and discovered remdesivir, ribavirin, galidesivir, and tenofovir is a powerful suppressor of RdRP enzymes, with restricting the value of energies between −7.0 to −7.8 kcal/mol [14].

Toremifene is an example of a viral inhibitor drug based on target repurposing. Martin and Cheng initially found toremifene as a possible COVID-19 drug molecule, followed by docking methodology up to spot the toremifene target molecules. They are successful with known 2 effective targets, particularly the spike-conjugated protein and NSP14 [15].

Artificial Intelligence-Based

Artificial intelligence (AI) and network medicine are cutting-edge applications of information science that define disease, medicine, treatments, and target identification with the least amount of error in the big data era. During this pandemic, artificial intelligence (AI)-based medicine repositioning has been highlighted globally. It was made potential by AI models and algorithms' tremendous computer capacity in processing and analyzing huge volumes of data of virulent disease and health care data [16]. Since then, academics have progressively leveraged this technology to my huge numbers of patient data and drug clinical trial records for data observation, with AI methods such as deep learning construction and graph depiction learning being deployed [17].

Worldwide research works are presently in progress to apply artificial intelligence-based medication repurposing for Coronavirus, which has been improved with the help of web servers and assets. While simulated intelligence medication repositioning is in its earliest stages, a few reports have shown empowering results. For example, utilizing Benevolent AI's information diagram, Richardson and collaborators distinguished baricitinib as likely helpful for COVID-19 from a rundown of supported medications [18]. To speed up the screening of drug libraries, AI can be employed in conjunction with other computational methodologies. In two independent investigations, for example, AI and molecular docking were used to find prospective COVID- 19 medicines [19].

Pathway-Based and Genetic Associations

During this pandemic, pathway mapping is a critical component of drug repositioning. As prospective gene targets discovered by genome-wide association studies (GWAS) may not be entirely accessible as therapeutic targets, this technique is critically important in GWAS data. Pathway study of genes upstream and or downstream of a GWAS-linked target may be employed in these situations to find attractive candidate medications for repurposing opportunities [20]. Knowledge, such as data on the expression of genes, interactions of protein, and metabolic pathways, are utilized in pathway mapping to build drug and illness networks and identify potential drug repurposing targets based on shared biological mechanisms.

The rise of genome-wide association studies (GWAS) over the last decade has resulted in a better understanding of the aetiology of numerous infectious diseases and the genetic variants linked to them. With the increasing availability of biological data, it is now feasible to find new targets for clinically licensed medications to address disease phenotypes investigated by GWAS, resulting in drug-reusing. Using GWAS, progress has been made in understanding the genetic variables implicated in the development of COVID-19. The Severe COVID-19 GWAS community found the 3p21.31 cluster of genes as a genetic risk locus in COVID-19-suffering patients with respiratory system failure in a GWAS research encompassing 1980 seriously ill COVID-19 patients. SLC6A20, LZTFL1, CCR9, FYCO1, CXCR6, and XCR1 are among the genes found on 3p21.31, and they could be new therapeutic targets for COVID-19 [21].

Experimental Approaches

Targeted Based Approaches

In this type of virtual screening, the potency of medications is determined by their ability to suppress a single target that is important for any disease multiplication, usually a gene protein [1]. Due to the simpler requirements, target-based screening is used in many drug repurposing studies. Xia *et al.* targeted the spike protein, *i.e.*, SARS-CoV-2 glycoprotein, which causes cell-cell fusion and arbitrates entrance of the virus into the host cell, in their drug repurposing study [22].

SARS-CoV-2 Drug Repurposing

Whereas not strictly a medication repurposing method, animal models have shown to be useful in the search for new COVID-19 treatment medicines. Ferrets, Syrian hamsters, mice, and primates, excluding humans, are among the numerous therapeutically relevant animal models that are frequently used to capture disease development *in vivo* [23]. In this section, researchers concentrate on the transgenic model of mice and the primates excluding humans, *i.e.*, non-human primate (NHP) paradigm. Bao and colleagues used hACE2 transgenic mice as a therapeutically compatible SARS-CoV-2 infection animal model [24]. ICR mice that have human ACE2 receptor proteins were used to create hACE2 transgenic mice, allowing for precise *in vivo* SARS-CoV-2 spike protein recapitulation and interaction with receptors of human ACE2. hACE2 mice infected with SARS-CoV-2 showed loss of weight and somewhat bristled hair, unlike wild-type mice, according to the research. In addition, the viral load in the hACE2 mice lungs was effectively identified by RT-qPCR. After that, the infectious COVID-19 virus was effectively recovered from the infected lung of hACE2 mice, proposing that the receptor protein of ACE2 is required for the entrance SARS-CoV-2 virus into the host cell. Furthermore, this work supported Koch's Postulate by demonstrating that SARS-CoV-2 is the causal agent of COVID-19 [1].

Drug Repurposing Molecules for COVID-19

Remdesivir

Remdesivir is an analogue of adenosine prodrug having a substituent of the nitrile group at the first position′, which confirmed broad-spectrum antibody with high potency in *in vitro* against a group of viruses consisting of MERS-CoV, COVID-19 virus, and Ebola virus [24 - 27]. Remdesivir evolved as an anti-Hepatitis-C Virus (HCV) candidate. Remdesivir turned into in addition examined in opposition to Ebola in medical trials, though its improvements were stopped because of the dearth of marked potency.

Many clinical trials centred on the potentially active remdesivir used for the therapy of coronavirus disease [28]. Hepatocellular toxicity, nausea, anaemia, renal damage, hypotension, respiratory failure, and constipation are among the mild to moderate side effects of remdesivir [29, 30]. Nonetheless, recent evidence supports the safe mode of administration of COVID-19 drug remdesivir to patients in hospitals. Remdesivir (Fig. **1**) is the first medicine approved by the FDA for the treatment of the disease of SARS-CoV-2 in adult human and child patients over the age of 12 who require hospitalization on May 1, 2020 [31]. Remdesivir was granted conditional approval in Europe on July 3, 2020, in the interests of public health and based on data that it satisfies a required medical need [32].

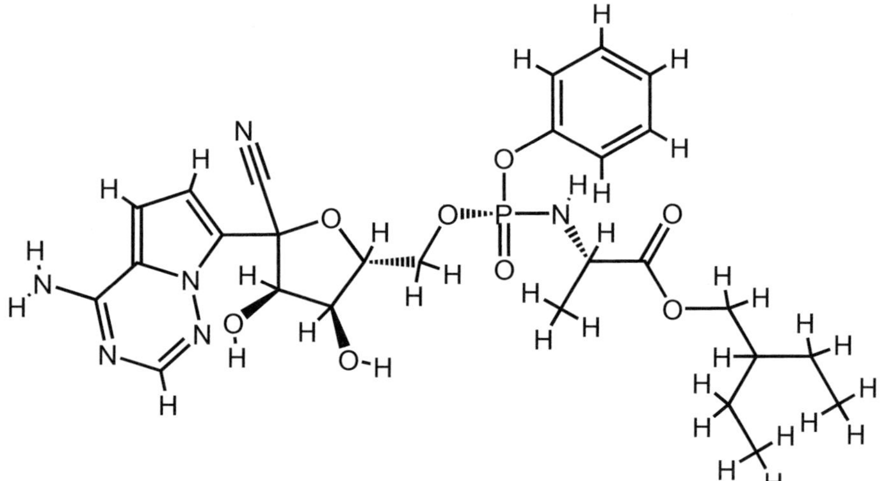

Remdesivir

Fig. (1). Structure of remdesivir.

Ribavirin

Ribavirin (Fig. **2**) mimics ATP and GTP with virus protein RNA-dependent RNA polymerase (RdRp) [33]. A cohort of ninety-four sufferers displayed that a mixture of IFN-α, lopinavir and or ritonavir, and ribavirin can additionally be helpful to sufferers of COVID-19 infection [34]. Other open-label, randomized, second-stage trials estimated the potency of IFN-β-1b mixture, lopinavir and or ritonavir, and ribavirin in curing patients infected with SARS-CoV-2. The triple remedy that used to be foremost to solely the use of lopinavir and or ritonavir in phases of curing patients with moderate or average COVID-19 infection. Yet, there are no scientific trials that without delay to assess the potency of ribavirin. Besides literature reports, there is other continuing research on a clinical trial of the COVID-19 drug through an aggregate of nitazoxanide, ribavirin, and ivermectin [35].

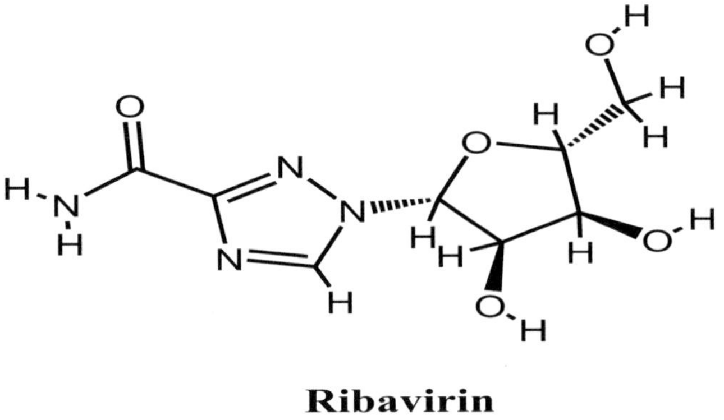

Fig. (2). Structure of Ribavirin.

Darunavir

Darunavir (Fig. **3**) is a protease inhibitor that was developed to treat the Human Immunodeficiency Virus (HIV) (HIV) [36]. Darunavir's efficacy in treating SARS-CoV-2 has not been tested in clinical studies. Riva *et al.* propose that darunavir at an 800mg/dose cannot protect HIV patients against COVID-19 infection and cannot care for patients of HIV from deteriorating pulmonary function caused by COVID-19, this report is based on case studies of three SARS-CoV-2 patients that already had an HIV infection [37]. Darunavir's effectiveness and safety are being evaluated in one current clinical study (NCT04252274) [35].

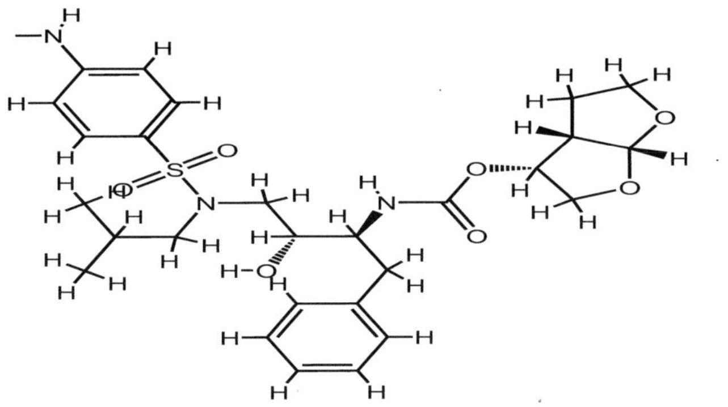

Darunavir

Fig. (3). Structure of Darunavir.

Chloroquine

For many years, chloroquine (Fig. **4**) has been used as an antimalaria medication. Its antiviral mechanism is unknown; however, studies show that it interferes with glycosylation of cell membrane receptor, and angiotensin-converting enzyme-2 (ACE2) of humans and hence impairs virus receptor interaction. According to recent research, the viral entry mechanism requires not just the spike protein of SARS-CoV-2 to bind to ACE2 and ganglioside, but chloroquine disrupts this process by fighting with the spike protein of the virus for ganglioside binding [38]. In a letter, Gao *et al.* said that clinical studies have shown that chloroquine outperforms control therapy in improving clinical outcomes in COVID-19 infected individuals [39]. The clinical trials, however, were not mentioned in the letter. Chloroquine phosphate therapy was shown to considerably shorten illness duration when compared to ritonavir lopinavir treatment in a controlled trial of 22 individuals. However, large-scale research is still needed to evaluate chloroquine's efficacy.

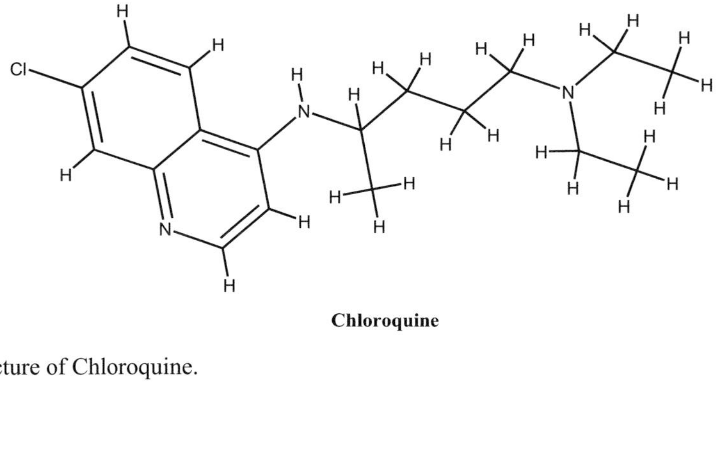

Chloroquine

Fig. (4). Structure of Chloroquine.

Hydroxychloroquine

The hydroxylated derivative of chloroquine, hydroxychloroquine (Fig. **5**), has antiviral properties comparable to chloroquine. In limited studies, hydroxychloroquine was proven to be beneficial for moderate COVID-19 therapy. The use of hydroxychloroquine, for example, was shown to considerably reduce the illness course in a randomized controlled study with 62 patients [40]. Another pilot factual research in a cohort of 80 moderately infected individuals found that taking hydroxychloroquine and azithromycin in combination may help infected patients [41]. However, when the same medicines and dosages were used to treat 11 individuals who were severely infected with COVID, another research found no significant clinical improvement. In a letter, it was stated that clinical investigations have shown that chloroquine is more effective than placebo [39]. COVID-19 infected individuals' clinical results improved after therapy. The letter, on the other hand, didn't provide any information on the clinical trials specifics. In a controlled trial of 22 individuals, it was discovered that, when compared to ritonavir/lopinavir, Chloroquine phosphate therapy decreased the length of the illness substantially [42]. Chloroquine and hydroxychloroquine have been linked to severe cardiac rhythm difficulties, blood and lymph system abnormalities, renal damage, and liver problems and failure, according to the FDA, which has advised against using these medicines outside of hospital settings [35].

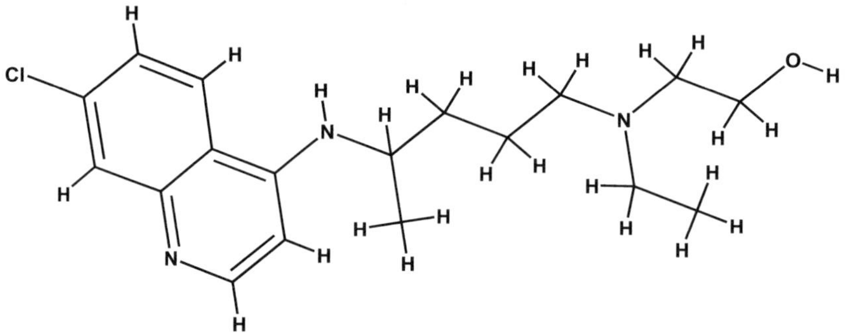

Hydroxychloroquine

Fig. (5). Structure of Hydroxychloroquine.

Dexamethasone

Dexamethasone (Fig. **6)** is a synthetic corticosteroid approved by FDA that inhibits the body's immune system by decreasing naïve T-cell division and differentiation and is used to treat immunological-related problems as first-line therapy [43]. Dexamethasone decreases the death percentage by one-third in patients getting the invasive blowing state of oxygen and one-fifth of patients were getting oxygen but not invasive blowing state of oxygen, according to a randomized, open-label trial including 6425 patients [44]. It does not affect the death rate in patients who do not require oxygen. A little rise in the level of blood glucose, ocular hypertension and cataract, side effects neuropsychology such as a change in behaviour and mood change [45], and are all metabolic side effects of dexamethasone. However, these side effects are more commonly linked with long-term high-dose dexamethasone therapy, whereas the benefit-risk balance for short-term therapies is favourable [46, 47]. Dexamethasone is being added to the COVID-19 therapeutic recommendations by the WHO.

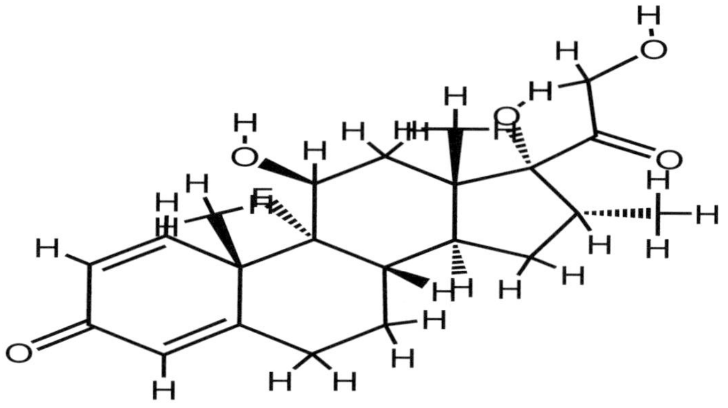

Dexamethasone

Fig. (6). Structure of Dexamethasone.

Emapalumab and Sarilumab

Sarilumab is an enemy of interleukin-6Ra (IL-6Rα) monoclonal antibodies (MoAb) endorsed for tolerable-to-extreme rheumatoid arthritis (RA) [48] with a clear-cut job additionally in obstructing IL-6 activity in disease [49], though emapalumab, coordinated with interferon-γ (IFN-γ), is utilized in the treatment of hemophagocytic lymphohistiocytosis [50] and is utilized with anakinra, an IL-1R enemy, in RA patients. Additionally, sarilumab and emapalumab can adequately balance the enormous cytokine discharge similar to COVID-19 virus contamination. Agenzia Italiana del Farmaco (AIFA) endorsed the utilization of each sarilumab or emapalumab in stage II and III clinical investigations, including hospitalized patients with Coronavirus pneumonic entanglements, to balance the cytokine storm [51].

Computational Study

Recently, the computational study of drugs using various software and algorithm, we can reuse the drug on another disease. This study includes molecular docking, molecular dynamic simulation and other virtual screen techniques. All these techniques require receptor and or ligand structure. A three-dimensional model of NSP10/NSP16 methyltransferase (PDB-ID: 6w61) and main protease (PDB-ID: 6lu7) of SARS-CoV-2 was used to perform virtual screening with a library of anti-viral, inti-infectious, and anti-protease compounds. It was observed that protease complexed with Cyclocytidine hydrochloride (anti-viral and anti-cancer), Trifluridine (anti-viral), Adonitol, and Meropenem (anti-bacterial), and Penciclovir (anti-viral) bound with a good docking score ranging from −6.8 to −5.1 (Kcal/mol). And NSP10/NSP16 methyltransferase complexed with Telbivudine, Oxytetracycline dihydrate (anti-viral), Methylgallate (anti-malarial), 2-deoxyglucose and Daphnetin (anti-cancer) from the docking score of −7.0 to −5.7 (Kcal/mol) [52]. To Identify a potent inhibitor of Methyltransferase, Endoribonuclease, Phosphatase and Main Protease enzymes of SARS-CoV-2 using coumarin derivatives, an *in silico* approach was performed. The top five ligands of each protein were taken, which showed good docking results for Methyltransferase, Endoribonuclease, Phosphatase and Main Protease and the top five compounds of each have docking scores from –9.00 to –7.97, –8.42 to –6.80, –8.63 to –7.48 and –7.30 to –6.01 kcal/mol, respectively. The docked compounds were further validated through MD simulation [53].

CONCLUSION

Drug repurposing is a field of medication research whose significance has been expanding in the past few years, because of a few benefits, like the probability to abbreviate the clinical preliminaries, the augmentation of the existence of an old medication by tracking down another remedial objective, and the disclosure of often ambiguous connections among evidently far off illnesses. The criticalness to discover medications to confront the Coronavirus pandemic has enormously caused this sort of examination in the past months. Computational methodologies have played and still assume an important part to look through weapons compelling against SARS-CoV-2 infections among the munitions build-up of medicines accessible today, yet until now, the output doesn't come to satisfy hopes. According to the researcher, an important job in this test of skill and capacity was played by basic bioinformatics, whose contributions were made believable additionally by the exceptional speed with which the constructions of the main coronavirus proteins were made available. However, many aftereffects of these examinations seem not completely satisfying. Many tests on a similar objective combined with the same medications do not give a certain proof of an impact. Besides, many experiments anticipate the adequacy of talked about drugs that neglected to show their adequacy in clinical preliminaries.

In this study, we sum up and accentuate the model reaction of mainstream researchers to the Coronavirus pandemic, which is remarkably adding to the effective repurposing of accessible medications. Antiviral specialists, for example, remdesivir, which turned into the primary medication explicitly supported to disable the replication of SARS-CoV-2 and adjunctive medications, LMWH and corticosteroids demonstrated profoundly viable in diminishing the death rate and the chance to recuperation in extreme/basic Coronavirus patients. In expansion, various trial drugs incorporating tocilizumab are accessible with regard to clinical preliminaries. The pandemic started short of what one year before the time this survey was composed, which firmly underlines the achievement and the quick responsiveness of the medication repurposing technique. In any case, a few endeavours should be spent in the improvement of strong and profoundly compelling antiviral medications and antibodies, for expanding the degree of readiness toward conceivable future pestilences.

CONSENT FOR PUBLICATION

Not applicable.

CONFLICT OF INTEREST

The authors declare no conflict of interest, financial or otherwise.

ACKNOWLEDGEMENTS

The authors thank the ministry of education government of India for providing a research fellowship and the Indian Institute of Information Technology Allahabad for providing us with Lab support and infrastructure.

REFERENCES

[1] Ng YL, Salim CK, Chu JJH. Drug repurposing for COVID-19: Approaches, challenges and promising candidates. Pharmacol Ther 2021; 228: 107930. [http://dx.doi.org/10.1016/j.pharmthera.2021.107930] [PMID: 34174275]

[2] https://www.who.int/emergencies/diseases/novel-coronavirus-2019

[3] https://www.who.int/director-general/speeches/detail/who-director-general-s-opening-remark--at-the-media-briefing-on-COVID-19---11-march-2020

[4] Rosa SGV, Santos WC. Clinical trials on drug repositioning for COVID-19 treatment. Rev Panam Salud Publica 2020; 44: 1. [http://dx.doi.org/10.26633/RPSP.2020.40] [PMID: 32256547]

[5] Velavan TP, Meyer CG. The COVID□19 epidemic. Trop Med Int Health 2020; 25(3): 278-80. [http://dx.doi.org/10.1111/tmi.13383] [PMID: 32052514]

[6] Kifle ZD, Ayele AG, Enyew EF. Drug repurposing approach, potential drugs, and novel drug targets for COVID-19 treatment. J Environ Public Health 2021; 2021: 1-11. [http://dx.doi.org/10.1155/2021/6631721] [PMID: 33953756]

[7] Sultana J, Crisafulli S, Gabbay F, Lynn E, Shakir S, Trifirò G. Challenges for drug repurposing in the COVID-19 pandemic era. Front Pharmacol 2020; 11: 588654. [http://dx.doi.org/10.3389/fphar.2020.588654] [PMID: 33240091]

[8] Cheng F. *In silico* oncology drug repositioning and polypharmacology. Methods Mol Biol. 2019; 1878: pp. 243-61.
[http://dx.doi.org/10.1007/978-1-4939-8868-6_15]

[9] Cheng F, Hong H, Yang S, Wei Y. Individualized network-based drug repositioning infrastructure for precision oncology in the panomics era. Brief Bioinform 2016; 18(4): 682-97.
[http://dx.doi.org/10.1093/bib/bbw051] [PMID: 27296652]

[10] Santos R, Ursu O, Gaulton A, *et al.* A comprehensive map of molecular drug targets. Nat Rev Drug Discov 2017; 16(1): 19-34.
[http://dx.doi.org/10.1038/nrd.2016.230] [PMID: 27910877]

[11] Pushpakom S, Iorio F, Eyers PA, *et al.* Drug repurposing: progress, challenges and recommendations. Nat Rev Drug Discov 2019; 18(1): 41-58.
[http://dx.doi.org/10.1038/nrd.2018.168] [PMID: 30310233]

[12] Abo-zeid Y, Ismail NSM, McLean GR, Hamdy NM. A molecular docking study repurposes FDA approved iron oxide nanoparticles to treat and control COVID-19 infection. Eur J Pharm Sci 2020; 153: 105465.
[http://dx.doi.org/10.1016/j.ejps.2020.105465] [PMID: 32668312]

[13] Li Q, Shah S. Structure-based virtual screening. In: Wu CH, Arighi CN, Ross KE, Eds. Protein Bioinformatics. New York, NY: Springer New York 2017; pp. 111-24.http://link.springer.com/10.1007/978-1-4939-6783-4_5 [Internet]
[http://dx.doi.org/10.1007/978-1-4939-6783-4_5]

[14] Elfiky AA. Ribavirin, Remdesivir, Sofosbuvir, Galidesivir, and Tenofovir against SARS-CoV-2 RNA dependent RNA polymerase (RdRp): A molecular docking study. Life Sci 2020; 253: 117592.
[http://dx.doi.org/10.1016/j.lfs.2020.117592] [PMID: 32222463]

[15] Martin WR, Cheng F. Repurposing of fda-approved toremifene to treat COVID-19 by blocking the spike glycoprotein and nsp14 of sars-cov-2. J Proteome Res 2020; 19(11): 4670-7.
[http://dx.doi.org/10.1021/acs.jproteome.0c00397] [PMID: 32907334]

[16] Cheng F, Desai RJ, Handy DE, *et al.* Network-based approach to prediction and population-based validation of *in silico* drug repurposing. Nat Commun 2018; 9(1): 2691.
[http://dx.doi.org/10.1038/s41467-018-05116-5] [PMID: 30002366]

[17] Zhou Y, Wang F, Tang J, Nussinov R, Cheng F. Artificial intelligence in COVID-19 drug repurposing. Lancet Digit Health 2020; 2(12): e667-76.
[http://dx.doi.org/10.1016/S2589-7500(20)30192-8] [PMID: 32984792]

[18] Richardson P, Griffin I, Tucker C, *et al.* Baricitinib as potential treatment for 2019-nCoV acute respiratory disease. Lancet 2020; 395(10223): e30-1.
[http://dx.doi.org/10.1016/S0140-6736(20)30304-4] [PMID: 32032529]

[19] Ton AT, Gentile F, Hsing M, Ban F, Cherkasov A. Rapid identification of potential inhibitors of sars-cov-2 main protease by deep docking of 1. 3 billion compounds. Mol Inform 2020; 39(8): 2000028.
[http://dx.doi.org/10.1002/minf.202000028] [PMID: 32162456]

[20] Mousavi SZ, Rahmanian M, Sami A. A connectivity map-based drug repurposing study and integrative analysis of transcriptomic profiling of SARS-CoV-2 infection. Infect Genet Evol 2020; 86: 104610.
[http://dx.doi.org/10.1016/j.meegid.2020.104610] [PMID: 33130005]

[21] Ellinghaus D, Degenhardt F, Bujanda L, *et al.* The Severe COVID-19 GWAS Group. Genomewide association study of severe COVID-19 with respiratory failure. N Engl J Med 2020; 383(16): 1522-34.
[http://dx.doi.org/10.1056/NEJMoa2020283] [PMID: 32558485]

[22] Xia S, Liu M, Wang C, *et al.* Inhibition of SARS-CoV-2 (previously 2019-nCoV) infection by a highly potent pan-coronavirus fusion inhibitor targeting its spike protein that harbors a high capacity to mediate membrane fusion. Cell Res 2020; 30(4): 343-55.

[http://dx.doi.org/10.1038/s41422-020-0305-x] [PMID: 32231345]

[23] Bao L, Deng W, Huang B, *et al.* The pathogenicity of SARS-CoV-2 in hACE2 transgenic mice. Nature 2020; 583(7818): 830-3. [http://dx.doi.org/10.1038/s41586-020-2312-y] [PMID: 32380511]

[24] Takayama K. *In vitro* and animal models for sars-cov-2 research. Trends Pharmacol Sci 2020; 41(8): 513-7. [http://dx.doi.org/10.1016/j.tips.2020.05.005] [PMID: 32553545]

[25] Warren TK, Jordan R, Lo MK, *et al.* Therapeutic efficacy of the small molecule GS-5734 against Ebola virus in rhesus monkeys. Nature 2016; 531(7594): 381-5. [http://dx.doi.org/10.1038/nature17180] [PMID: 26934220]

[26] Sheahan TP, Sims AC, Graham RL, *et al.* Broad-spectrum antiviral GS-5734 inhibits both epidemic and zoonotic coronaviruses. Sci Transl Med 2017; 9(396): eaal3653. [http://dx.doi.org/10.1126/scitranslmed.aal3653] [PMID: 28659436]

[27] Agostini ML, Andres EL, Sims AC, Graham RL, Sheahan TP, Lu X, *et al.* Coronavirus Susceptibility to the Antiviral Remdesivir (GS-5734) Is Mediated by the Viral Polymerase and the Proofreading Exoribonuclease. mBio 2018; 9(2). https://journals.asm.org/doi/10.1128/mBio.00221-18

[28] Burki TK. Completion of clinical trials in light of COVID-19. Lancet Respir Med 2020; 8(12): 1178-80. [http://dx.doi.org/10.1016/S2213-2600(20)30460-4] [PMID: 33010809]

[29] Humeniuk R, Mathias A, Cao H, Osinusi A, Shen G, Chng E, *et al.* Safety, tolerability, and pharmacokinetics of remdesivir, an antiviral for treatment of covid-19, in healthy subjects. Clin Transl Sci 2020. 5;cts. 12840. [http://dx.doi.org/10.1111/cts.12840]

[30] Elsawah HK, Elsokary MA, Abdallah MS, ElShafie AH. Efficacy and safety of remdesivir in hospitalized Covid-19 patients: Systematic review and meta-analysis including network meta-analysis. Rev Med Virol 2021; 31(4): e2187.https://onlinelibrary.wiley.com/doi/10.1002/rmv.2187 [http://dx.doi.org/10.1002/rmv.2187] [PMID: 33128490]

[31] https://www.fda.gov/news-events/press-announcements/coronavirus-COVID-19-update-fda-issues-emergency-use-authorization-potential-COVID-19-treatment

[32] 2020.https://www.ema. europa.eu/en/medicines/human/EPAR/veklury#authorisationdetails-

[33] Gordon CJ, Tchesnokov EP, Woolner E, *et al.* Remdesivir is a direct-acting antiviral that inhibits RNA-dependent RNA polymerase from severe acute respiratory syndrome coronavirus 2 with high potency. J Biol Chem 2020; 295(20): 6785-97. [http://dx.doi.org/10.1074/jbc.RA120.013679] [PMID: 32284326]

[34] Hung IFN, Lung KC, Tso EYK, *et al.* Triple combination of interferon beta-1b, lopinavir–ritonavir, and ribavirin in the treatment of patients admitted to hospital with COVID-19: an open-label, randomised, phase 2 trial. Lancet 2020; 395(10238): 1695-704. [http://dx.doi.org/10.1016/S0140-6736(20)31042-4] [PMID: 32401715]

[35] Wang X, Guan Y. COVID-19 drug repurposing: A review of computational screening methods, clinical trials, and protein interaction assays. Med Res Rev 2021; 41(1): 5-28. [http://dx.doi.org/10.1002/med.21728] [PMID: 32864815]

[36] Spagnuolo V, Castagna A, Lazzarin A. Darunavir for the treatment of HIV infection. Expert Opin Pharmacother 2018; 19(10): 1149-63. [http://dx.doi.org/10.1080/14656566.2018.1484901] [PMID: 29913082]

[36] Riva A, Conti F, Bernacchia D, *et al.* Darunavir does not prevent SARS-CoV-2 infection in HIV patients. Pharmacol Res 2020; 157: 104826. [http://dx.doi.org/10.1016/j.phrs.2020.104826] [PMID: 32325127]

[38] Fantini J, Di Scala C, Chahinian H, Yahi N. Structural and molecular modelling studies reveal a new mechanism of action of chloroquine and hydroxychloroquine against SARS-CoV-2 infection. Int J Antimicrob Agents 2020; 55(5): 105960. [http://dx.doi.org/10.1016/j.ijantimicag.2020.105960] [PMID: 32251731]

[39] Gao J, Tian Z, Yang X. Breakthrough: Chloroquine phosphate has shown apparent efficacy in treatment of COVID-19 associated pneumonia in clinical studies. Biosci Trends 2020; 14(1): 72-3. [http://dx.doi.org/10.5582/bst.2020.01047] [PMID: 32074550]

[40] Chen Z, Hu J, Zhang Z, Jiang S, Han S, Yan D, *et al.* Efficacy of hydroxychloroquine in patients with COVID-19: results of a randomized clinical trial 2020; 2020.03.22.20040758.https:// www.medrxiv.org/content/10.1101/2020.03.22.20040758v3 Internet [http://dx.doi.org/10.1101/2020.03.22.20040758]

[41] Gautret P, Lagier JC, Parola P, *et al.* Clinical and microbiological effect of a combination of hydroxychloroquine and azithromycin in 80 COVID-19 patients with at least a six-day follow up: A pilot observational study. Travel Med Infect Dis 2020; 34: 101663. [http://dx.doi.org/10.1016/j.tmaid.2020.101663] [PMID: 32289548]

[42] Huang M, Tang T, Pang P, Li M, Ma R, Lu J, *et al.* Treating COVID-19 with Chloroquine In: J Wu, Ed. Journal of Molecular Cell Biology. 2020; 18: pp. (12(4))322-5.

[43] Giles AJ, Hutchinson M-KND, Sonnemann HM. Dexamethasone-induced immunosuppression: mechanisms and implications for immunotherapy. j immunotherapy cancer. 2018 Dec;6(1):51.

[44] Horby P, Lim WS, Emberson J, Mafham M, Bell J, Linsell L, *et al.* Effect of dexamethasone in hospitalized patients with COVID-19 – preliminary report 2020; 2020.06.22.20137273.https:// www.medrxiv.org/content/10.1101/2020.06.22.20137273v1 Internet [http://dx.doi.org/10.1101/2020.06.22.20137273]

[45] Fassbender Adeniran JM, Jusufbegovic D, Schaal S. Common and rare ocular side-effects of the dexamethasone implant. Ocul Immunol Inflamm 2017; 25(6): 834-40. [http://dx.doi.org/10.1080/09273948.2016.1184284] [PMID: 27379861]

[46] MIT, Centre for Biomedical Engineering, 500 Technology Square, Cambridge, MA, 02139, USA, Black R, Grodzinsky A. Dexamethasone: chondroprotective corticosteroid or catabolic killer? eCM. 2019 Nov 22;38:246–63 .

[47] Q&A: dexamethasone and COVID-19. 2020 [Internet]. [cited 2021 Oct 7]. Available from: https://www.who.int/news-room/q-a-detail/q-a-dexamethasone-and-COVID-19

[48] Huizinga TWJ, Fleischmann RM, Jasson M, *et al.* Sarilumab, a fully human monoclonal antibody against IL-6Rα in patients with rheumatoid arthritis and an inadequate response to methotrexate: efficacy and safety results from the randomised SARIL-RA-MOBILITY Part A trial. Ann Rheum Dis 2014; 73(9): 1626-34. [http://dx.doi.org/10.1136/annrheumdis-2013-204405] [PMID: 24297381]

[49] Kampan NC, Xiang SD, McNally OM, Stephens AN, Quinn MA, Plebanski M. Immunotherapeutic interleukin-6 or interleukin-6 receptor blockade in cancer: challenges and opportunities. Curr Med Chem 2018; 25(36): 4785 806. [http://dx.doi.org/10.2174/0929867324666170712160621] [PMID: 28707587]

[50] Al-Salama ZT. Emapalumab: first global approval. Drugs 2019; 79(1): 99-103. [http://dx.doi.org/10.1007/s40265-018-1046-8] [PMID: 30623346]

[51] Clinical Trials - COVID-19 [Internet]. [cited 2021 Oct 7]. Available from: https://www.aifa.gov.it/sperimentazioni-cliniche-COVID-19

[52] Maurya SK, Maurya AK, Mishra N, Siddique HR. Virtual screening, ADME/T, and binding free energy analysis of anti-viral, anti-protease, and anti-infectious compounds against NSP10/NSP16 methyltransferase and main protease of SARS-CoV-2. J Recept Signal Transduct Res 2020; 40(6): 605-12.

[http://dx.doi.org/10.1080/10799893.2020.1772298] [PMID: 32476594]

[53] Maurya AK, Mishra N. *In silico* validation of coumarin derivatives as potential inhibitors against Main Protease, NSP10/NSP16-Methyltransferase, Phosphatase and Endoribonuclease of SARS-CoV-2. J Biomol Struct Dyn 2021; 39(18): 7306-21. [http://dx.doi.org/10.1080/07391102.2020.1808075] [PMID: 32835632]

CHAPTER 8

Virtual Screening of Phytochemicals in Search of a Potential Drug Candidate for COVID-19: DFT Study and Molecular Docking

Nikita Tiwari[1,*], **Lubna Jamal**[1] and **Anil Mishra**[1]

[1] *Department of Chemistry, University of Lucknow, Lucknow-226007, Uttar Pradesh, India*

Abstract: The global health pandemic due to COVID-19 caused by SARS-CoV-2, affected and changed the world's condition drastically. Herein, we evaluated the bioactivity of some phytochemicals as inhibitors against SARS-CoV-2 M provirus (6LU7) using computational models. We reported the optimization of phytochemicals employing density functional theory (DFT) with B3LYP/6-311G+(d,p) level theory. DFT calculations were employed to determine the free energy, dipole moment as well as chemical reactivity descriptors. Molecular docking has been performed against the SARS-CoV-2 M provirus to search the binding affinity and interactions of all compounds with the respective protein. The known drug, Chloroquine of SARS-CoV-2 main protease, was also docked to evaluate its binding affinity. Besides, the data from DFT, the docking studies predicted that flavonoids (Quercetin, Myricetin, Apigenin and Daidzein) have the least binding affinity and might serve as a potent inhibitor against SARS-CoV-2 comparable with the approved medicine, Chloroquine. The high binding affinity of flavonoids was attributed to the presence of hydrogen bonds along with different hydrophobic interactions between the flavonoid and the critical amino acid residues of the receptor. The DFT calculations showed that flavonoids have high-lying HOMO, electrophilicity index and dipole moment. All these parameters could share a different extent to significantly affect the binding affinity of these phytochemicals with active protein sites.

Keywords: Apigenin, B3LYP, Chloroquine, COVID-19, DFT Calculations, Daidzein, Dipole Moment, Electrophilicity Index, Flavonoids, HOMO, Hydrogen Bonds, Hydrophobic Interactions, Molecular Docking, Myricetin, Pandemic, Phytochemicals, Quercetin, SARS-CoV-2.

INTRODUCTION

In the final month of the year 2019, a major cluster of strange pneumonia due to a novel coronavirus was reported in Wuhan metropolis, China [1]. Despite efforts to

* **Corresponding author Nikita Tiwari:** Department of chemistry, Lucknow University, Lucknow-226007, Uttar Pradesh, India: E-mail: nikitalko23@gmail.com

Tahmeena Khan & Alfred J. Lawrence (Eds.)

include the outbreak inside the preliminary place, the dissemination of SARS-CoV-2 has continued to spread widely to different countries. Therefore, in March 2020, the WHO declared the uncontrollable spread of SARS- CoV-2 as a pandemic [2]. Now, after more than two years after the initiation of the infection, this disease is still a threat to human life [3]. The control of SARS- CoV-2 is the need of the hour not only for human health but also for the prosperity of the nations and the betterment of society, and to achieve this purpose, global collaborations are very important [4].

Coronavirus (CoV), the virus responsible for COVID-19, belongs to the family Coronaviridae. They have spikes on their surfaces and contribute to a huge group of viruses containing RNA genome [5]. Based on the genetic and serological relationship, the coronaviruses are broadly classified into four major groups- Alpha, Beta, Gamma and Delta [6]. These RNA viruses are mainly distributed among birds and mammals [7] and have a very high potential to infect the human respiratory system [7, 8]. HCoV-OC43, -229E, -NL63, -HKU1, SARS-CoV (Severe Acute Respiratory Syndrome – Coronavirus), MERS-CoV (Middle East Respiratory Syndrome – Coronavirus) and now SARS-CoV-2 are a few examples of coronaviruses that infect humans [6, 9].

In the search for the cure, complete knowledge of the cause is pretty much important. Cryogenic electron microscopic studies and many other studies show that SARS-CoV-2 binds to the cell membrane of ACE2 (Angiotensin-converting enzyme 2) [10, 11]. The genome of coronavirus carries two replicase polyproteins that undergo proteolytic processing into a set of mature NSP (non-structural proteins) that function during viral replication, including RdRp, 3CL-Mpro, Papain-like proteinase (PL2pro) and a superfamily 1-like helicase (HEL1) [12]. According to the structure, the genome of SARS-CoV-2 (novel coronavirus) encodes many important proteins for its replication in the host genome, such as M (membrane protein), S(spike protein), N (nucleocapsid protein), E (envelop protein) and coronavirus main protease. These proteins play a pivotal role in gene expression and cleave polyproteins into replication-related proteins [13, 14]. The structure of 3CL-Mpro comprises three domains, *i.e.*, I, II and III, where domains I and II are N-terminal domains while domain III is a C-terminal domain [15].

To control and cure the SARS-CoV-2 infection, drug designing and development of the vaccine are necessary. Nowadays, many researchers around the globe are involved in studying chemicals with anti-viral properties. Many naturally occurring phytochemicals have anti-viral effects and pharmacological properties [16]. According to the ancient Indian texts 'SUSHRUT SAMHITA' and 'CHARAK SAMHITA' ancient people used the different parts of plants to cure themselves of various infectious diseases [17, 18]. *Toona sinensis* [18, 19],

Jatropha curcas [18, 20], *Glycyrrhiza glabra* [18, 21], *Daucas carota* [18, 22], *Piper chaba* [18, 23], *Cinnamomum zeylanicum* [18, 24], *Zingiber officinale* [18, 25], *etc.* are some common plants that are used to treat the diseases since ancient times, or we can say that their therapeutic uses are well known. Different parts of these plants contain a large number of phytochemicals (Table **1**), and the medicinal properties of these phytochemicals provide them with a very special place in the field of drug design or medicinal research. So we can say that phytochemicals may provide potential solutions to the SARS-CoV-2 pandemic.

The inhibition property of phytochemicals is related to their ability to inhibit the virus from attaching to the 3CL-Mpro [29, 30]. In this work, we studied certain phytochemicals (*apigenin, benzoic acid, daidzein, furfural, furfuryl formate, gallic acid, 4- hydroxybenzoic acid, maltol, oxalic acid, pyragallol, salicylic acid, succinic acid, 2,3-butanediol, propionic acid, eugenol, cinnamaldehyde, caffeic acid, pentanol, piperonal, 2,3,5-trymethyl pyrazine, asparagine, quercetin, mercytin)* to understand their utility in drug designing and effectiveness against SARS-CoV-2 *via* DFT calculations and molecular docking. Molecular docking is a robust, effective, low-cost and less time-consuming process than traditional drug discovery methods [31]. *Chloroquine* is taken as a reference compound for this study.

Table 1. Plants and their constituent chemicals active against virus diseases.

Plants	Plant Image	Family	Part Used	Chemicals
Jatropha curcas	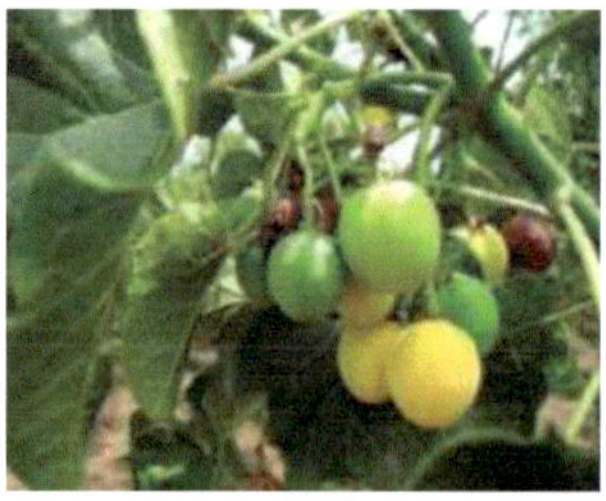 [26]	Euphorbiaceae	Leaves, Latex	Apigenin, benzoic acid, daidzein, pyragallol, salicylic acid, gallic acid
Glycyrrhiza glabra	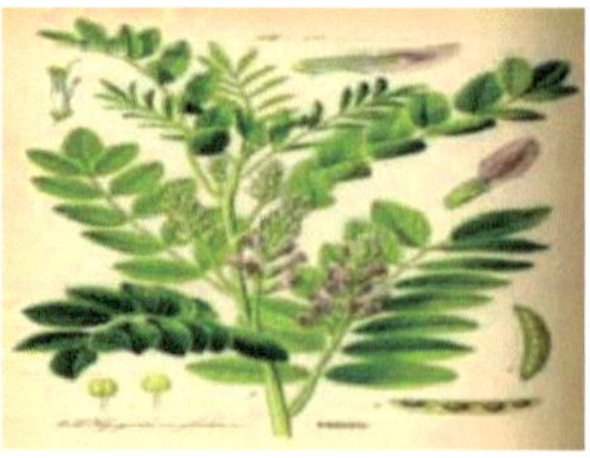 [27]	Leguminosae	Root	Pentanol, furfural, Furfuryl formate, maltol, butanediol, propionic acid

(Table 1) cont.....

Plants	Plant Image	Family	Part Used	Chemicals
Daucas Carota	-	Apiaceae	Root	Caffeic acid, flavonoids
Piper Chaba	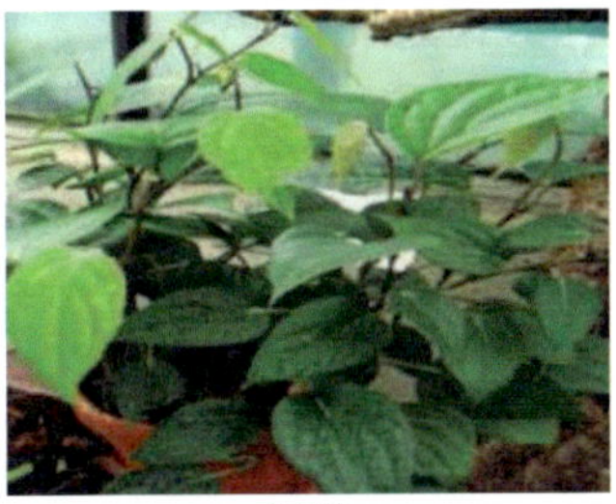 [23]	Piperaceae	Leaves, Stem bark	Piperanol
Cinnamomum zeylanicum	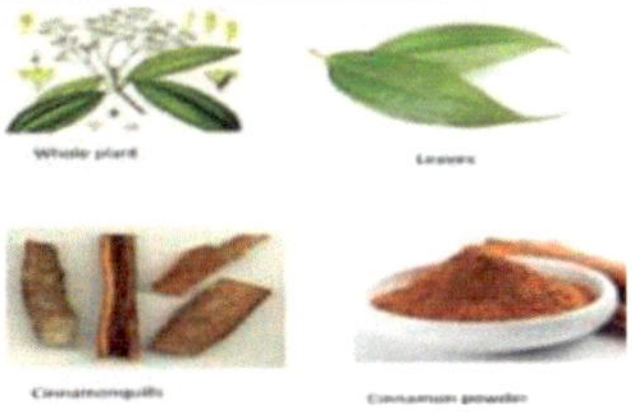 [24]	Lauraceae	Bark, Leaves, whole plant	Cinnamaldehyde, Eugenol
Zingiber officinale	-	Zingiberaceae	Rhizome, Root	Oxalic acid
Toona sinensis	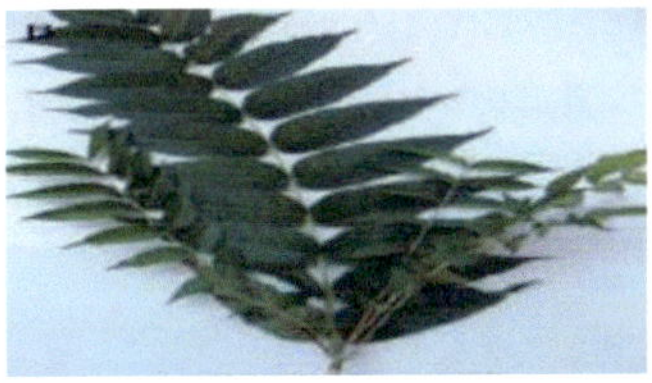 [28]	Meliaceae	Leaves	Gallic acid, Quercitin

MATERIALS AND METHODS

DFT Calculations

In this study, computational calculations were done using the DFT level of theory with the hybrid functional B3LYP using 6-311G+(d, p) basis set in the gas phase in the Gaussian09 programme package [32]. The study starts with the optimization of the geometry of all the phytochemicals, and then the optimized geometrical parameters are used in the calculation of the energy of HOMO (Highest Occupied Molecular Orbital), LUMO (Lowest Unoccupied Molecular Orbital), energy gap (ΔE), dipole moment (μ) and free energy. The initial geometry of phytochemicals was taken from an online chemical information resource named PubChem and further modified in Gaussian 09 software using GaussView5 [33]. The absence of imaginary frequency confirmed that phytochemicals were fully optimized. Chemical reactivity descriptors such as hardness (η), softness (δ), electronegativity (χ) and electrophilicity index (ω) of all the phytochemicals were also calculated from the energies of frontier HOMOs and LUMOs. The equations used for the calculations of reactivity descriptors have been reported in our earlier publications [34, 35].

Molecular Docking

The three-dimensional crystal structure of the SARS-CoV-2 M provirus (PDB ID: 6LU7) was retrieved in PDB format from an online protein data bank (PDB) [36]. All the present hetero atoms along with water molecules, were removed, and the energy minimization of the protein was implemented by Auto dock 4.2 software [37]. Then optimized phytochemicals were subjected to a molecular docking study against SARS-CoV-2 M provirus (6LU7). In computer-aided drug design, binding affinity and mode(s) of the ligand with the target protein can predict by molecular docking simulation. Finally, molecular docking simulation was performed by Auto dock Tools considering the protein as a macromolecule and the phytochemical as a ligand. In this study, rigid docking was performed where all rotatable bonds were converted into non-rotatable ones with the centre grid box size -26.346, 12.605, and 58.919 Å along x, y and z directions, respectively. The number of points in the x, y and z directions are 126, 126 and 126, respectively. After docking, both the protein and ligand structures were saved in. pdbqt format required to analyze and visualize the docking result and search the interactions between ligands and amino acid residues of the receptor protein. The results were shown using Ligplot.

RESULT AND DISCUSSION

DFT Calculation Studies

The DFT calculations were undertaken using Gaussian09 software at B3LYP 6-311G+(d,p) basis set. The optimized structures (Fig. **1**) of the phytochemicals were drawn with Gauss View 5.

Thermodynamic Properties

The thermodynamic properties, such as free energy, are important to predict the stability of any given chemical reaction. Greater negative values indicate improved thermodynamic properties. This study found that the values are negative (Table **2**), meaning the binding will occur spontaneously without any extra energy expenditure. The free energy of Chloroquine is -1326.289 Hartree, whereas flavonoids show similar energy, which suggests that the molecules are energetically and configurationally more preferable. The dipole moment of Chloroquine is 7.113 Debye, where flavonoids show a near about dipole moment to the chloroquine. The elevated level of dipole moment enhances the hydrogen bond formation, nonbonding interaction, binding affinity and polar nature of a molecule.

Chloroquine 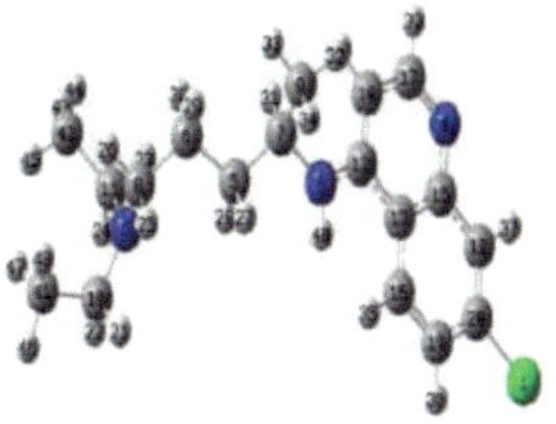	**Apigenin** 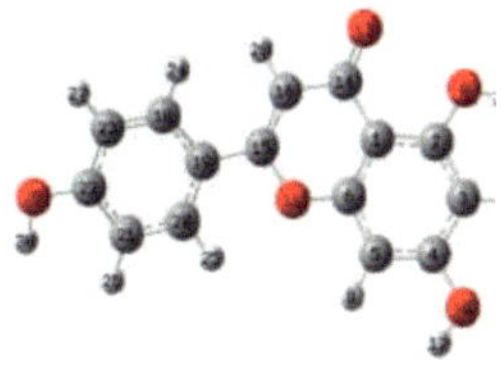	**Benzoic acid** 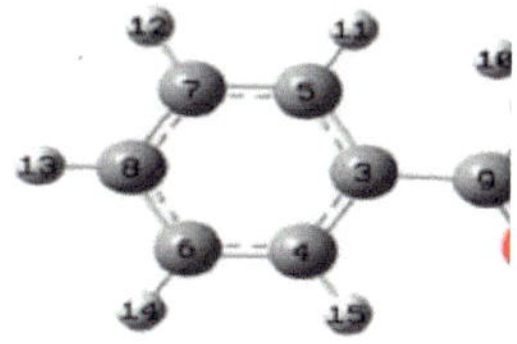
Diadzein 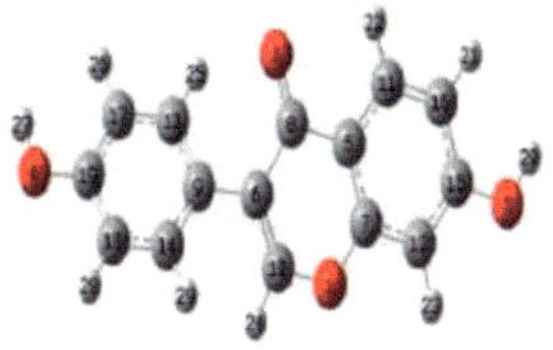	**Furfural** 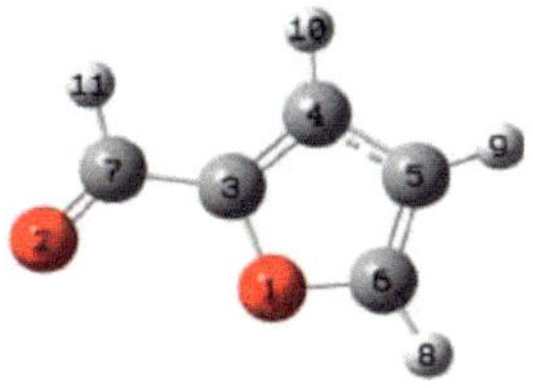	**Furfuryl formate** 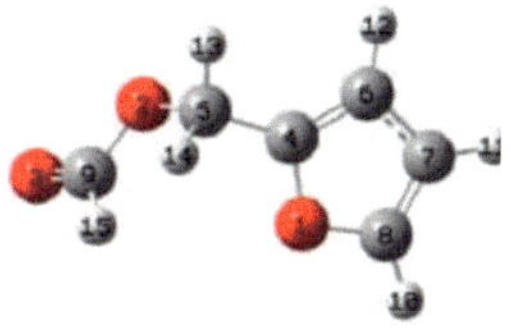
Gallic acid 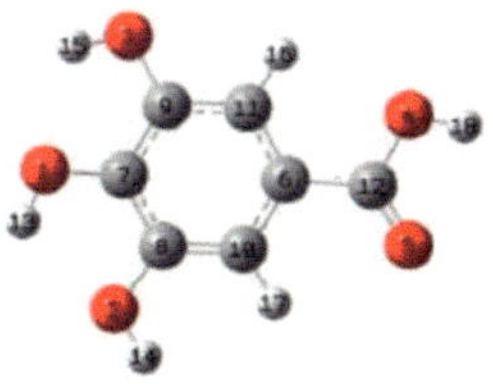	**4-Hydroxybenzoic acid** 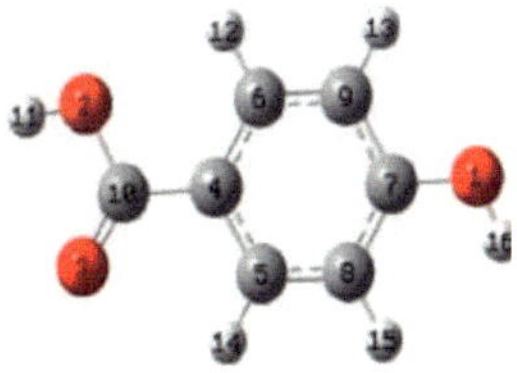	**Maltol** 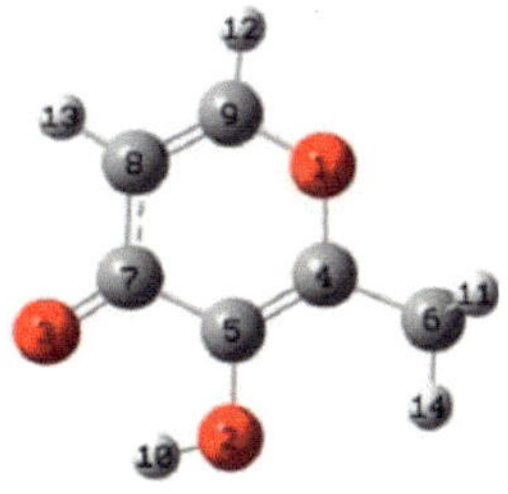
Oxalic acid 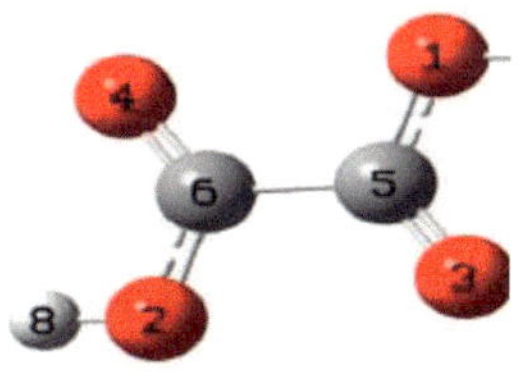	**Pyrogallol** 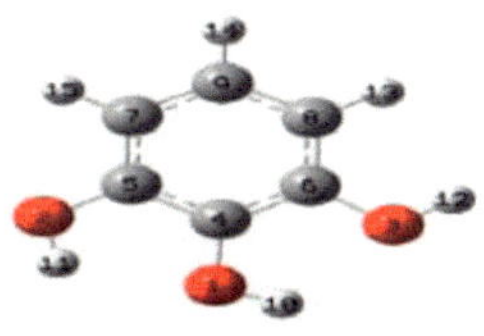	**Salicylic acid** 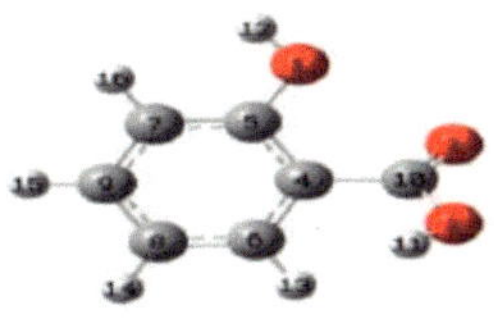
Succinic acid	**2,3-Butanediol**	**Propionic acid**

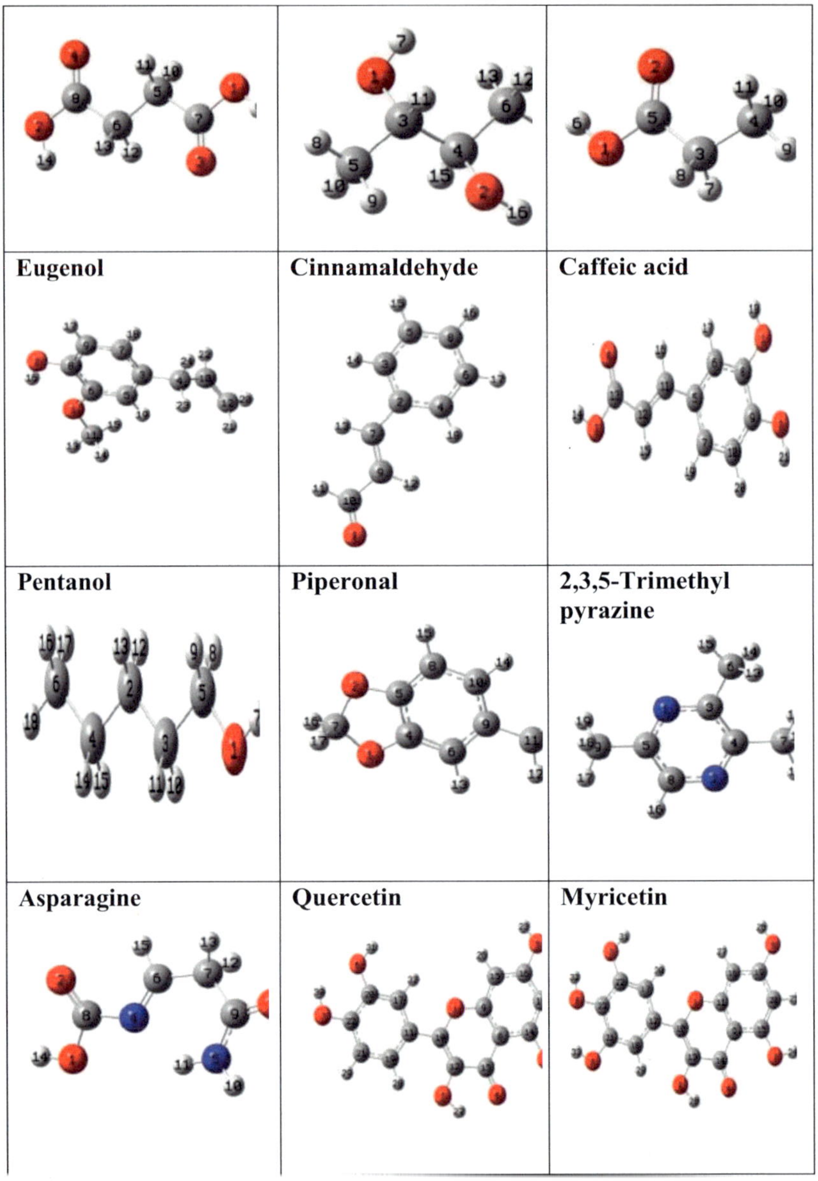

Fig. (1). The optimized structure of investigated phytochemicals and chloroquine.

Table 2. Free energy (in Hartree) and dipole moment (Debye) of chloroquine and all the phytochemicals.

Ligand	Free Energy	Dipole Moment
Chloroquine	-1326.289	7.113
Apigenin	-953.994	6.586

(Table 2) cont.....

Ligand	Free Energy	Dipole Moment
Benzoic acid	-420.937	5.050
Diadzein	-878.748	2.332
Furfural	-343.446	4.521
Furfuryl formate	-458.020	4.845
Gallic acid	-646.694	2.344
4-Hydroxybenzoic acid	-496.197	1.926
Maltol	-458.039	3.702
Oxalic acid	-378.448	0.051
Pyrogallol	-458.055	2.973
Salicylic acid	-496.178	5.784
Succinic acid	-457.112	3.002
2,3-Butanediol	-308.989	2.275
Propionic acid	-268.489	1.612
Eugenol	-538.856	2.643
Cinnamaldehyde	-423.092	4.917
Caffeic acid	-648.861	2.413
Pentanol	-273.067	1.623
Piperonal	-534.133	4.314
2,3,5-Trimethyl pyrazine	-382.381	0.649
Asparagine	-491.388	3.127
Quercetin	-1104.495	6.493
Myricetin	-1179.742	7.283

Molecular Orbital Properties

The hardness and softness of a molecule can be obtained from its energy gap, *i.e.*, the HOMO-LUMO gap. The large energy gap is related to high kinetic stability and low chemical reactivity, and the small energy gap represents low chemical stability because the addition of electrons to a higher LUMO and the withdrawal of electrons from a lower HOMO is energetically favourable in a certain reaction. In this analysis, Chloroquine has a HOMO-LUMO gap of 4.30 eV (Fig. **2**), where flavonoids Quercetin (3.74 eV) and Myricetin (3.77 eV) shows the lower energy gap and the lower chemical potential (-3.89 eV) with the highest chemical softness (0.53 eV) values as compared to the chloroquine which may contribute the higher chemical reactivity than others (Table **3**).

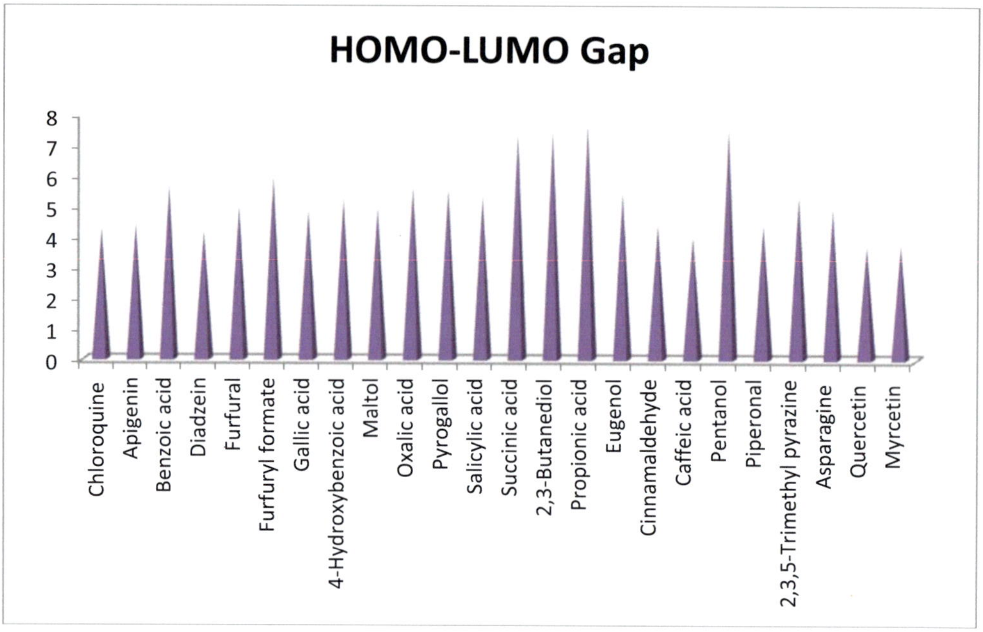

Fig. (2). Pictorial representation of energy gap (HOMO-LUMO gap) for all the investigated compounds.

Table 3. HOMO, LUMO, gap, hardness (η), softness (δ), electronegativity (χ), electrophilicity index (ω), ionization potential (I) and electron affinity (A) of all the compounds.

Ligand	HOMO	LUMO	ΔE	χ	η	δ	ω	I	A
Chloroquine	-5.81	-1.51	4.30	-3.66	2.15	0.46	3.11	5.81	1.51
Apigenin	-6.30	-1.85	4.45	-4.07	2.22	0.45	3.73	6.30	1.85
Benzoic acid	-7.63	-1.88	5.75	-4.75	2.87	0.34	3.93	7.63	1.88
Diadzein	-6.06	-1.85	4.21	-3.95	2.10	0.47	3.71	6.06	1.85
Furfural	-7.20	-2.15	5.05	-4.67	2.52	0.39	4.32	7.20	2.15
Furfuryl formate	-6.91	-0.92	5.99	-3.91	2.99	0.33	2.55	6.91	0.92
Gallic acid	-6.51	-1.61	4.90	-4.06	2.45	0.40	3.36	6.51	1.61
4-Hydroxybenzoic acid	-6.85	-1.57	5.28	-4.21	2.64	0.37	3.35	6.85	1.57
Maltol	-6.64	-1.66	4.98	-4.15	2.49	0.40	3.45	6.64	1.66
Oxalic acid	-8.16	-2.49	5.67	-5.32	2.83	0.35	5.00	8.16	2.49
Pyrogallol	-6.12	-0.51	5.61	-3.31	2.80	0.35	1.95	6.12	0.51
Salicylic acid	-6.92	-1.53	5.39	-4.22	2.69	0.37	3.31	6.92	1.53
Succinic acid	-8.07	-0.63	7.44	-4.35	3.72	0.26	2.54	8.07	0.63
2,3-Butanediol	-7.66	-0.18	7.48	-3.92	3.74	0.26	2.05	7.66	0.18

(Table 3) cont.....

Ligand	HOMO	LUMO	ΔE	χ	η	δ	ω	I	A
Propionic acid	-7.96	-0.23	7.73	-4.09	3.86	0.25	2.16	7.96	0.23
Eugenol	-5.86	-0.39	5.47	-3.12	2.73	0.36	1.78	5.86	0.39
Cinnamaldehyde	-6.95	-2.51	4.44	-4.73	2.22	0.45	5.03	6.95	2.51
Caffeic acid	-6.20	-2.16	4.04	-4.18	2.02	0.49	4.32	6.20	2.16
Pentanol	-7.60	-0.01	7.59	-3.80	3.79	0.26	1.90	7.60	0.01
Piperonal	-6.42	-1.98	4.44	-4.20	2.22	0.45	3.97	6.42	1.98
2,3,5-Trimethyl pyrazine	-6.78	-1.39	5.39	-4.08	2.69	0.37	3.09	6.78	1.39
Asparagine	-7.35	-2.39	4.96	-4.87	2.48	0.40	4.78	7.35	2.39
Quercetin	-5.76	-2.02	3.74	-3.89	1.87	0.53	4.04	5.76	2.02
Myricetin	-5.78	-2.01	3.77	-3.89	1.88	0.53	4.02	5.78	2.01

Binding Affinity and Binding Interactions Analysis

Docking simulation studies were done to predict the binding mode of phytochemicals at the SARS-CoV-2 M pro pocket (Fig. **3**). Similarly, the Chloroquine was docked in the protein pocket as a control. The binding affinity of phytochemicals ranged between -1.22 to -6.36 Kcal/mol. The results showed that flavonoids are located in the active pocket, similar to chloroquine. Chloroquine showed binding energy of -4.79 kcal/mol (Fig. **4**), whereas increasing order of binding energy followed the sequence such as Myricetin<Quercetin<Apigenin<Daidzein (-5.49<-5.68<-5.8<-6.36) kcal/mol. Except for ordinary hydrogen bonding, nonbonding interactions have frequently used the term to determine the shape and behaviour of molecules. From molecular docking analysis, the major and common residues of 6LU7 active sites like HIS163, CYS145, MET165, THR190, HIS164, LEU167, GLU166, GLN189 and PRO168 form different significant interactions with the ligands (Table **4**).

Table 4. Binding affinity and non-binding interactions of all the investigated compounds.

Ligand	Binding Energy	Interacting Amino Acids
Chloroquine	-4.79	HIS163, CYS145, MET165, THR190, HIS164, LEU167, GLU166, GLN189, PRO168
Apigenin	-5.8	HIS163, CYS145, GLU166, GLN189, MET165, ASP187, ARG188, HIS41, HIS164, LEU141 (2.92 Å), SER144 (2.84 Å)
Benzoic acid	-3.76	ARG4, PHE291, LEU282, TRP207, PHE3, GLU288, LYS5 (3.16 Å)
Daidzein	-6.36	GLU166, MET165, ASP187, ARG188, MET49, GLN189, HIS164, HIS163, LEU141, CYS145 (3.04 Å), PHE140 (3.07 Å)

(Table 4) cont.....

Ligand	Binding Energy	Interacting Amino Acids
Furfural	-3.28	HIS164, MET165, ARG188, TYR54, GLN189, MET49, HIS41, PRO52, ASP187
Furfuryl formate	-2.95	PRO52, MET49, ARG188, MET165, GLN189, HIS41, ASP187, TYR54 (2.92 Å)
Gallic acid	-2.74	PHE219, GLU270, LEU271, TRP218, ASN221 (3.26 Å), ARG279 (2.71 Å), GLY275 (2.87 Å)
4-Hydroxybenzoic acid	-3.77	ARG4, GLU288, PHE291, LEU282, PHE3, LYS5 (3.13 Å), TRP207 (2.72 Å)
Maltol	-3.32	LEU75, VAL77, ARG76, GLN74, PHE66, LEU67, HIS64 (2.63 Å)
Oxalic acid	-1.64	VAL303, GLY302 (3.05 Å), SER1 (2.85 Å & 3.19 Å)
Pyrogallol	-3.04	ASN63, HIS64, ARG76, LEU67, GLN74 (3.26 Å), PHE66 (2.94 Å & 2.99 Å), VAL77 (2.77 Å & 3.03 Å)
Salicylic acid	-3.6	LYS5, ARG4, PHE291, LEU282, SER284, GLU288, TRP207, PHE3 (3.03 Å)
Succinic acid	-1.22	HIS80, LYS90, GLY79, VAL35, LYS88, SER81
2,3-Butanediol	-2.27	PHE3, TRP207, SER284, GLU288, LEU282 (2.89 Å & 3.05 Å)
Propionic acid	-1.96	MET17, GLY15, GLU14 (3.02 Å), LYS97 (2.74 Å)
Eugenol	-4.36	MET165, TYR54, ASP187, MET49, GLN189, THR190, ARG188, GLU166 (3.04 Å & 3.32 Å)
Cinnamaldehyde	-4.19	MET165, GLN189, ASP187, HIS41, ARG188, HIS164, GLU166
Caffeic acid	-3.55	GLU288, PHE291, PHE3, ARG4, LYS5, SER284, LEU282, TRP207 (2.60 Å)
Pentanol	-2.61	PRO52, ARG188, MET165, HIS164, ASP187, GLN189, MET49, HIS41, TYR54 (2.72 Å)
Piperonal	-4.18	MET165, GLN189, HIS41, MET49, ASP187, ARG188, PRO52, TYR54, HIS164
2,3,5-Trimethyl pyrazine	-4.16	MET49, ARG188, HIS41, HIS164, MET165, TYR54, ASP187, PRO52
Asparagine	-2.79	ARG4, LYS5, PHE3, PHE291, LEU282, TRP207 (2.94 Å)
Quercetin	-5.68	HIS41, GLN189, MET165, GLU166, PRO168, LEU167, THR190, ARG188, TYR54 (2.77 Å), ASP187 (3.14 Å)
Myricetin	-5.49	HIS164, MET165, GLU166, PRO168, LEU167, ARG188, GLN189, HIS41 (3.31 Å), TYR54 (2.85 Å), THR190 (2.89 Å & 3.00 Å), ASP187 (3.02 Å), GLN192 (3.06 Å)
-	-	-
-	-	-

(Table 4) cont.....

Ligand	Binding Energy	Interacting Amino Acids
-	-	-
-	-	-
-	-	-
-	-	-
-	-	-
-	-	-

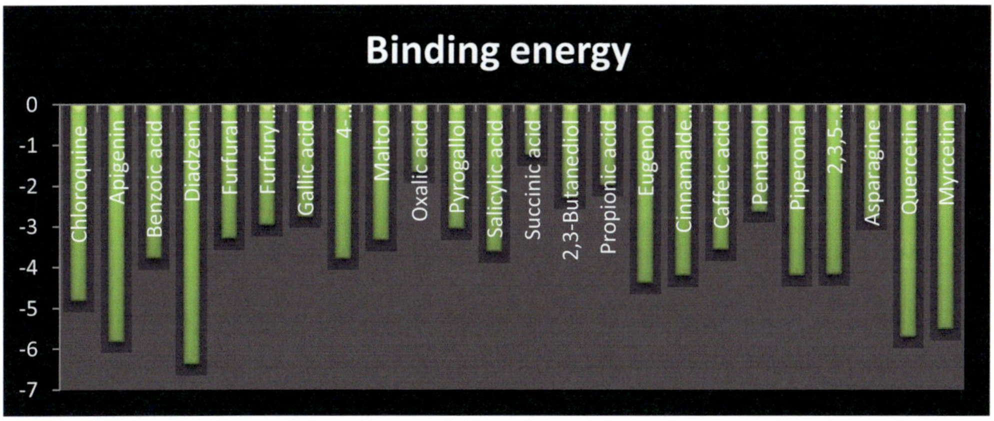

Fig. (3). Graphical representation of binding energies of all the selected compounds.

AutoDock results show that among all the phytochemicals(taken in this study), the binding affinities of apigenin(-5.8 kcal/mol), daidzein(-6.36 kcal/mol), quercetin(-5.68kcal/mol) and myricetin(-5.49 kcal/mol) is comparable to well-known ligand chloroquine(-4.79 kcal). Daidzein showed the lowest binding affinity and interacted hydrophobically with the residues GLU166, MET165, ASP187, ARG188, MET49, GLN189, HIS164, HIS163 AND LEU141. The polar interactions were found to be with Phe140(3.07 Å) and CYS 145(3.04 Å). Hydrogen bonding and different hydrophobic interactions between the inhibitor and the amino acid residues of the receptor are responsible for the binding affinity of daidzein. The result of the docking studies shows that the amino acid residue HIS163, CYS145, GLU166, GLN189, MET165, ASP187, ARG188, HIS41, and HIS164 interacted hydrophobically with the apigenin molecule, whereas LEU141(2.92 Å) and SER144(2.84 Å) show polar interactions. The phytochemical quercetin also shows good interaction with 3CL-Mpro. The hydrophobic interaction was found with residues HIS41, GLN189, MET165, GLU166, PRO168, LEU167, THR190 and ARG188; and hydrogen bonding with Tyr54(2.77 Å) and Asp187(3.14 Å). However, myricetin interacts hydrophobically with HIS164, MET165, GLU166, PRO168, LEU167, ARG188 and GLA189. Tyr54(2.85 Å), His41(3.31 Å), Asp187(3.02 Å), Gln192(3.06 Å) and Thr190(2.89 Å) show polar interactions. Hence, these phytochemicals have the potential to combat SARS-CoV-2.

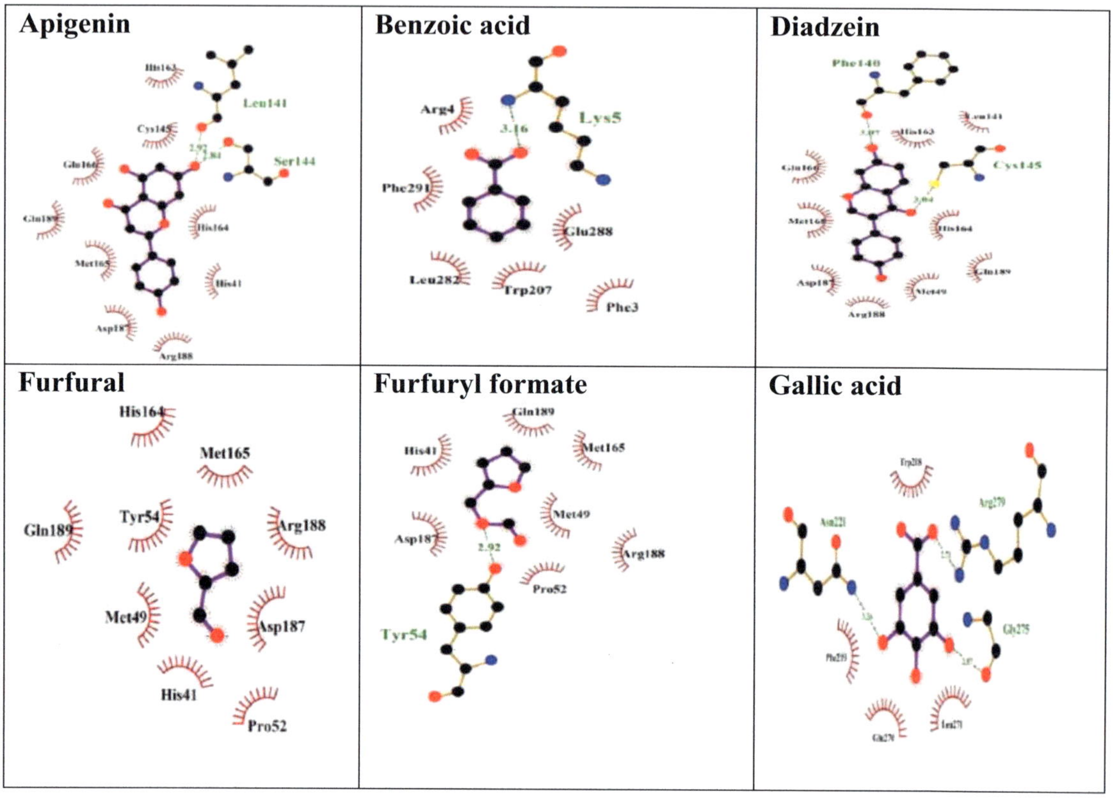

(Fig. 4) contd.....

4-Hydroxybenzoic acid

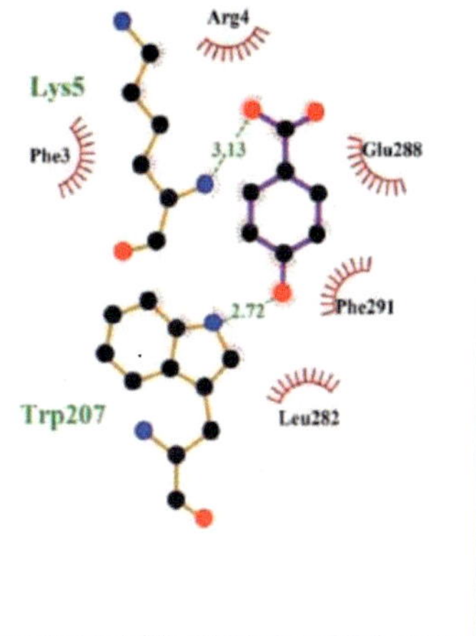

Maltol

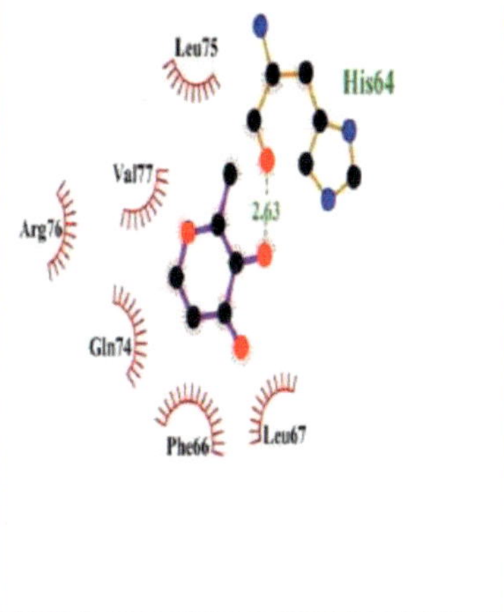

Oxalic acid

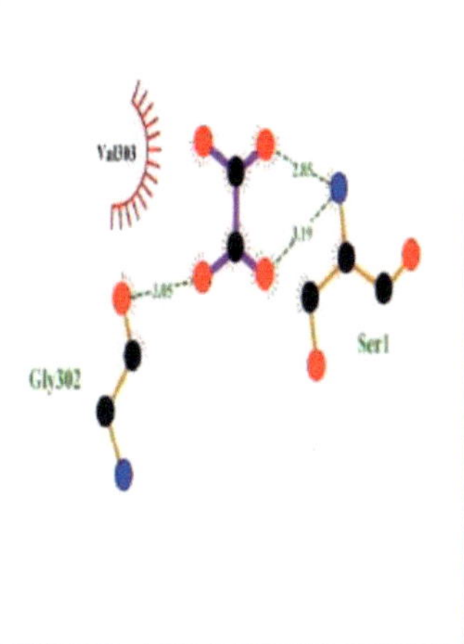

Pyrogallol

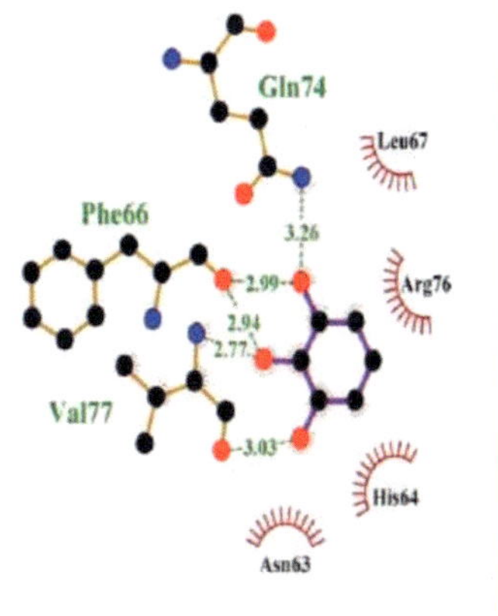

Salicylic acid

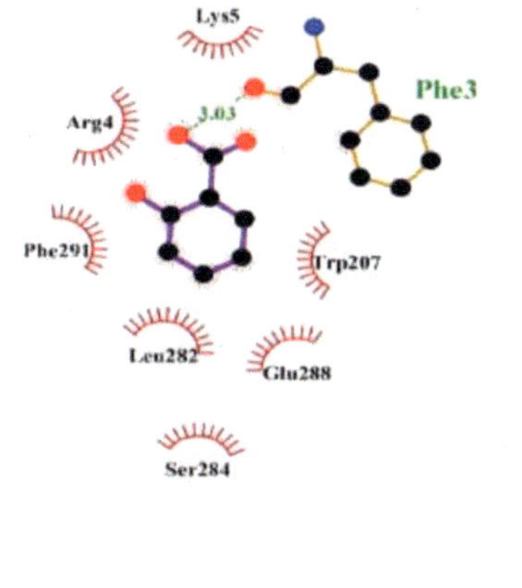

Succinic acid

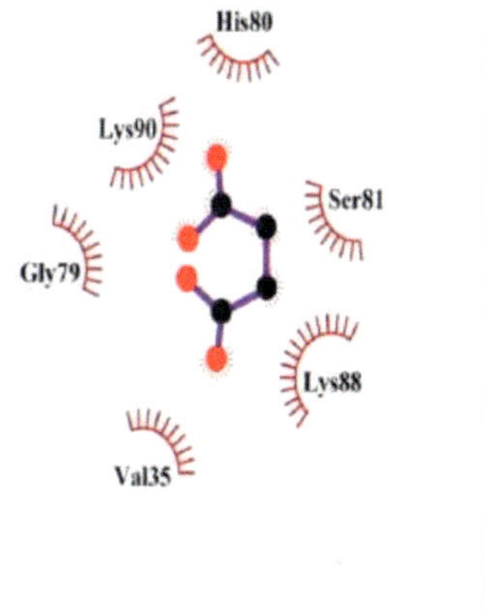

2,3-Butanediol

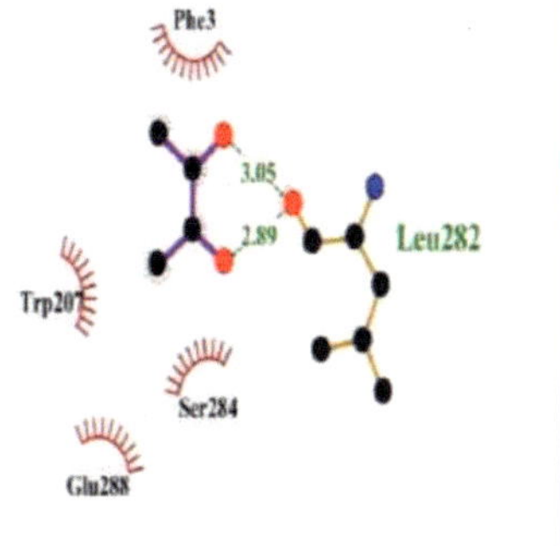

Propionic acid

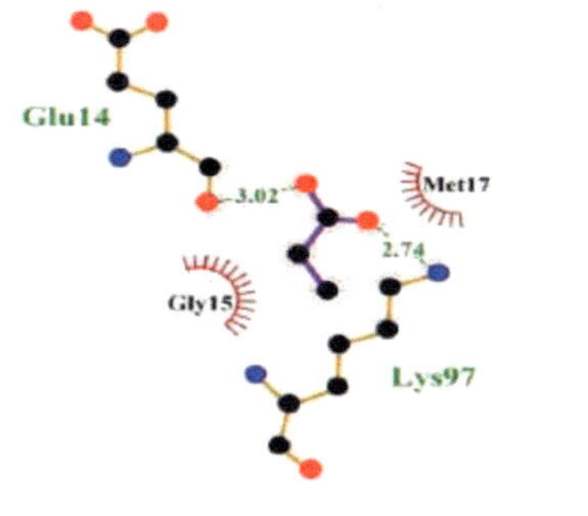

Eugenol

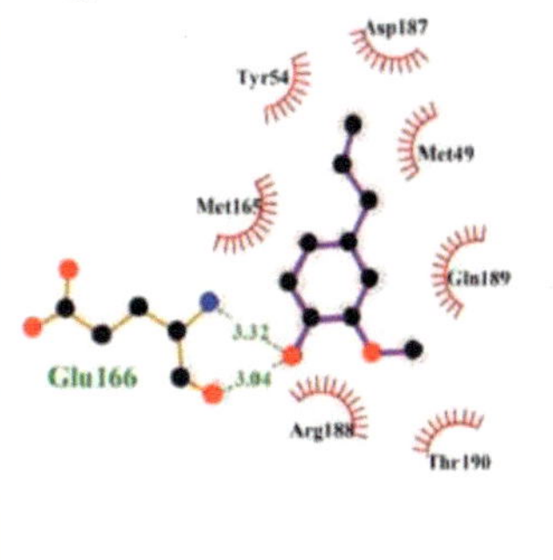

Cinnamaldehyde | **Caffeic acid** | **Pentanol**

(Fig. 4) contd.....

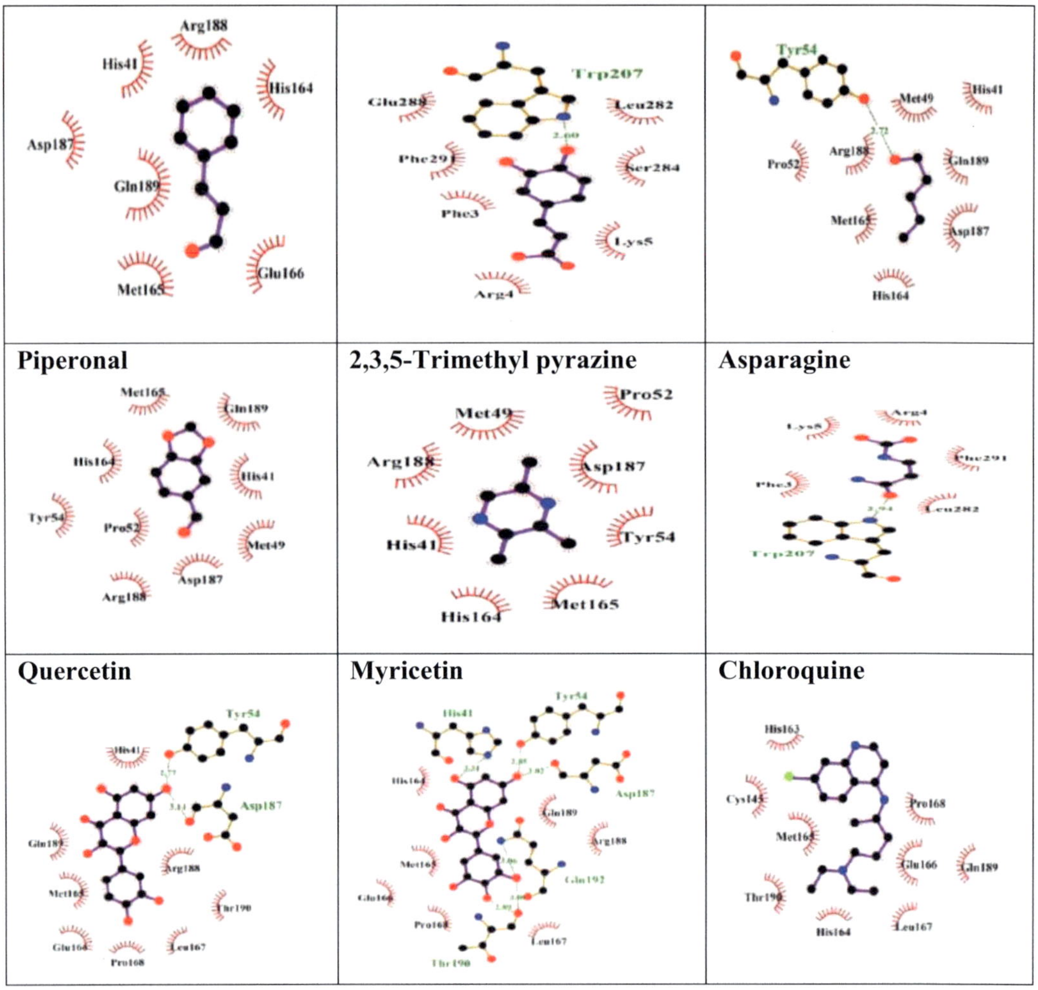

Fig. (4). Amino acid residues in the binding pocket of SARS-CoV-2 M pro involved in interactions with the phytochemicals and chloroquine.

CONCLUSION

In this study, the inhibitory action of phytochemicals against the SARS-CoV-2 M provirus has been studied. From the DFT calculations, all the compounds are thermally stable, and some (flavonoids) of them show better chemical reactivity than Chloroquine, a known drug. Among all the phytochemicals studied, Flavonoids show greater dipole moments with a smaller energy gap. The docking results also confirmed that flavonoids with lower binding affinities than chloroquine are more potent inhibitors against the SARS-CoV-2 M provirus. This study may be helpful in understanding the physicochemical and biological properties of phytochemicals against this novel coronavirus.

CONSENT FOR PUBLICATION

Not applicable.

CONFLICT OF INTEREST

The authors declare no conflict of interest, financial or otherwise.

ACKNOWLEDGEMENTS

The authors are thankful to the Central Facility for Computational Research (CFCR), University of Lucknow, for providing access to computational models throughout the work.

REFERENCES

[1] Wang Y, Wang Y, Chen Y, Qin Q. Unique epidemiological and clinical features of the emerging 2019 novel coronavirus pneumonia (COVID-19) implicate special control measures. J Med Virol 2020; 92(6): 568-76.
[http://dx.doi.org/10.1002/jmv.25748] [PMID: 32134116]

[2] Zhou P, Yang XL, Wang XG, *et al.* A pneumonia outbreak associated with a new coronavirus of probable bat origin. Nature 2020; 579(7798): 270-3.
[http://dx.doi.org/10.1038/s41586-020-2012-7] [PMID: 32015507]

[3] WHO coronavirus disease (COVID-19) dashboard. Geneva: World Health Organization 2021.

[4] Kaur SP, Gupta V. COVID-19 Vaccine: A comprehensive status report. Virus Res 2020; 288: 198114.
[http://dx.doi.org/10.1016/j.virusres.2020.198114] [PMID: 32800805]

[5] Peele KA, Potla Durthi C, Srihansa T, *et al.* Molecular docking and dynamic simulations for antiviral compounds against SARS-CoV-2: A computational study. Informatics in Medicine Unlocked 2020; 19: 100345.
[http://dx.doi.org/10.1016/j.imu.2020.100345] [PMID: 32395606]

[6] Corman VM, Muth D, Niemeyer D, Drosten C. Hosts and sources of endemic human coronaviruses. In: Advances in virus research.Elsevier Inc. 2018; 100: pp. 163-88.
[http://dx.doi.org/10.1016/bs.aivir.2018.01.001]

[7] Masters PS. The molecular biology of coronaviruses. Adv Virus Res 2006; 66(06): 193-292.
[http://dx.doi.org/10.1016/S0065-3527(06)66005-3] [PMID: 16877062]

[8] Spaan W, Cavanagh D, Horzinek MC. Coronaviruses: structure and genome expression. J Gen Virol 1988; 69(12): 2939-52.
[http://dx.doi.org/10.1099/0022-1317-69-12-2939] [PMID: 3058868]

[9] Andersen KG, Rambaut A, Lipkin WI, Holmes EC, Garry RF. The proximal origin of SARS-CoV-2. Nat Med 2020; 26(4): 450-2.
[http://dx.doi.org/10.1038/s41591-020-0820-9] [PMID: 32284615]

[10] Walls AC, Park YJ, Tortorici MA, *et al.* Structure, function, and antigenicity of the SARS-CoV-2 spike glycoprotein. Cell 2020; 180: 1-12.
[http://dx.doi.org/10.1016/j.cell.2020.02.058]

[11] Yang J, Roy A, Zhang Y. Protein–ligand binding site recognition using complementary binding-specific substructure comparison and sequence profile alignment. Bioinformatics 2013; 29(20): 2588-95.
[http://dx.doi.org/10.1093/bioinformatics/btt447] [PMID: 23975762]

[12] Cheng A, Zhang W, Xie Y, *et al.* Expression, purification, and characterization of SARS coronavirus RNA polymerase. Virology 2005; 335(2): 165-76.
[http://dx.doi.org/10.1016/j.virol.2005.02.017] [PMID: 15840516]

[13] Graham RL, Sparks JS, Eckerle LD, Sims AC, Denison MR. SARS coronavirus replicase proteins in pathogenesis. Virus Res 2008; 133(1): 88-100.
[http://dx.doi.org/10.1016/j.virusres.2007.02.017] [PMID: 17397959]

[14] Prasad A, Prasad M. SARS-CoV-2: the emergence of a viral pathogen causing havoc on human existence. J Genet 2020; 99(1): 37.
[http://dx.doi.org/10.1007/s12041-020-01205-x] [PMID: 32482926]

[15] Tassakka ACMAR, Sumule O, Massi MN, *et al.* Potential bioactive compounds as SARS-CoV-2 inhibitors from extracts of the marine red alga *Halymenia durvillei* (Rhodophyta) – A computational study. Arab J Chem 2021; 14(11): 103393.
[http://dx.doi.org/10.1016/j.arabjc.2021.103393] [PMID: 34909061]

[16] Perez RM. Antiviral activity of compounds isolated from plants. Pharm Biol 2003; 41(2): 107-57.
[http://dx.doi.org/10.1076/phbi.41.2.107.14240]

[17] Thakur S, Asrani RK, Patil RD, Thakur M. Antimicrobial potential of medicinal plants of Himachal Pradesh against pathogenic Escherichia Coli, Salmonella Gallinarum and Salmonella Typhimurium. Vet Res (Faisalabad) 2018; 6: 67-71.

[18] Pal S, Chowdhury T, Paria K, *et al.* Brief survey on phytochemicals to prevent COVID-19. J Indian Chem Soc 2022; 99(1): 100244.
[http://dx.doi.org/10.1016/j.jics.2021.100244]

[19] Chojnacka K, Witek-Krowiak A, Skrzypczak D, Mikula K, Młynarz P. Phytochemicals containing biologically active polyphenols as an effective agent against Covid-19-inducing coronavirus. J Funct Foods 2020; 73: 104146.
[http://dx.doi.org/10.1016/j.jff.2020.104146] [PMID: 32834835]

[20] Thomas R, Sah N, Sharma P. Therapeutic biology of Jatropha curcas: a mini review. Curr Pharm Biotechnol 2008; 9(4): 315-24.
[http://dx.doi.org/10.2174/138920108785161505] [PMID: 18691091]

[21] Hasan MK, Ara I, Mondal MSA, *et al.* Phytochemistry, pharmacological activity, and potential health benefits of Glycyrrhiza glabra. Heliyon 2021; e07240-7.
[http://dx.doi.org/10.1016/j.heliyon.2021.e07240]

[22] Al-Snafi PDAE. Nutritional and therapeutic importance of *Daucus carota*- A review. IOSR J Pharm 2017; 7(2): 72-88.
[http://dx.doi.org/10.9790/3013-0702017288]

[23] Haque ME, Roy AC, Rani M. Review on Phytochemical and Pharmacological Investigation of *Piper chaba* Hunter. Int J Sci Eng Res 2018; 9(3): 1.

[24] Mishra N, Srivastava R. Therapeutic and Pharmaceutical Potential of Cinnamon. Ethnopharmacological Investigation of Indian Spices 2020. In book: Ethnopharmacological Investigation of Indian Spices (pp.124-136).
[http://dx.doi.org/10.4018/978-1-7998-2524-1.ch010]

[25] Ghosh AK, Banerjee S, Mullick HI, *et al.* Zingiber officinale: A Natural Gold. Int J Pharma Bio Sci 2011; 2(1): 1.

[26] Abobatta W. Jatropha curcas: an overview. J Adv Agric 2019; 10: 1650-6.

[http://dx.doi.org/10.24297/jaa.v10i0.8145]

[27] Sharma V, Agrawal RC. *Glycyrrhiza glabra*- A Plant For The Future; Mintage J Pharm Med Sci 2008.

[28] Peng W, Liu Y, Hu M, *et al. Toona sinensis*: a comprehensive review on its traditional usages, phytochemisty, pharmacology and toxicology. Rev Bras Farmacogn 2019; 29(1): 111-24. [http://dx.doi.org/10.1016/j.bjp.2018.07.009] [PMID: 32287507]

[29] Muteeb G, Alshoaibi A, Aatif M, *et al.* Screening marine algae metabolites as high – affinity inhibitors of SARS – CoV – 2 main protease (3CLpro): an *in silico* analysis to identify novel drug candidates to combat COVID – 19 pandemic. Applied. Bioorg Chem 2020; 63(1): 1.

[30] Palese LL. The structural landscape of SARS-CoV-2 main protease: hints for inhibitor search. ChemRxiv 2020. [http://dx.doi.org/10.26434/chemrxiv.12209744.v1]

[31] Bharti R, Shukla SK. Molecules against Covid-19: An *in silico* approach for drug development. Journal of Electronic Science and Technology 2021; 19(1): 100095. [http://dx.doi.org/10.1016/j.jnlest.2021.100095]

[32] Frisch MJ, *et al.* Gaussian 09, Revision D01. Wallingford, CT: Gaussian, Inc. 2009.

[33] Dennington R, Keith T, Millam J. GaussView, version 5. Shawnee Mission, KS, USA: Semichem Inc. 2009.

[34] Tiwari N, Kumar A, Pandey A, Mishra A. Computational investigation of dioxin-like compounds as human sex hormone-binding globulin inhibitors: DFT calculations, docking study and molecular dynamics simulations. Comput Toxicol 2022; 21: 100198. [http://dx.doi.org/10.1016/j.comtox.2021.100198]

[35] Tiwari N, Pandey A, Kumar A, Mishra A. Computational models reveal the potential of polycyclic aromatic hydrocarbons to inhibit aromatase, an important enzyme of the steroid biosynthesis pathway. Comput Toxicol 2021; 19: 100176. [http://dx.doi.org/10.1016/j.comtox.2021.100176]

[36] Jin Z, Du X, Xu Y, *et al.* Structure of M^{pro} from SARS-CoV-2 and discovery of its inhibitors. Nature 2020; 582(7811): 289-93. [http://dx.doi.org/10.1038/s41586-020-2223-y] [PMID: 32272481]

[37] Morris GM, Huey R, Lindstrom W, *et al.* AutoDock4 and AutoDockTools4: Automated docking with selective receptor flexibility. J Comput Chem 2009; 30(16): 2785-91. [http://dx.doi.org/10.1002/jcc.21256] [PMID: 19399780]

CHAPTER 9

Role of Immunity Against COVID-19

Nidhi Singh[1,*]

[1] *Department of Chemistry, Isabella Thoburn College, Lucknow-226007, India;*

Abstract: The chapter defines the importance of immunity against COVID-19. The chapter describes the immunopathogenesis of COVID-19 and the way the body fights back and shows its immune response against the pathogen. Factors affecting immunity include ageing and obesity. The effect of the age factor has been visible in the suffering due to the coronavirus. The chapter also describes the nutritional factors that could boost immunity and enhance the immune response of the body against COVID-19. The major nutritional elements comprise vitamins and micronutrients, responsible for the biosynthesis of amino acids and strengthening of the defence system of the body. Natural products also play an important role in the enhancement of immunity against the coronavirus. The phytoconstituents present in plants play an active biochemical role in controlling COVID-19 symptoms. Vaccination has also helped in gaining acquired immunity against the COVID-19 pathogen and helped in developing herd immunity as well.

KEYWORDS: COVID-19, Immunity, Immunopathogenesis, Herd Immunity, Micronutrients, Phytoconstituents, Vaccination, Vitamins.

INTRODUCTION

Immunity is the natural defence system of human beings to protect them against various pathogenic diseases. Certain barriers evolved cell types, and antigen-antibody response relationships form the basis of human immunity. It is a response that is always active and is enhanced in times of infection. The importance of immunity is highly marked in our lives. A most recent example of this is being witnessed, as the world is in the clutches of coronavirus or COVID-19. The virus was named such, because of its initiation in the year 2019. It has been two years since then, and the virus continues to create havoc in the world. Various studies and reports have shown the importance or role of immunity during this pandemic [1, 2]. People with higher immunity have better survived this pandemic, rather than the ones with compromised immunity. It can be

* **Corresponding author Nidhi Singh:** Department of Chemistry, Isabella Thoburn College, Lucknow,-226007, India; E-mail: nidhi.singh23081993@gmail.com

Tahmeena Khan & Alfred J. Lawrence (Eds.)

witnessed through the case of children, who were least affected by this virus, as they had stronger immunity than elderly people. Since coronavirus came as a new virus variant and elderly people had no memorized or acquired immunity against it, they suffered the most as most of them had other comorbidities like diabetes, blood pressure, heart problems, or respiratory problems. Coronavirus effect combined with these morbidities proved fatal to many of them. The spread of the virus was also rapid, as there was no underlying immunity against this virus. Thus, it can be deduced that immunity plays an important role against the COVID-19 virus [3, 4].

Coronavirus causes an outbreak of severe acute respiratory disorder wherein the virus disrupts the functioning of respiration, causing heavy breathing and loss of breath. In acute cases, the patient needs to be shifted to a ventilator as the virus may gradually attack other organs as well, and the patient may die of multiple organ failure.

Immune System: Process and Defense

The immune system consists of natural and acquired immunity. Innate or natural immunity exists from birth, like barriers or first-line defence, while acquired immunity refers to immunity acquired over the years based on memorization of their antigen-antibody responses to pathogens [5]. The general functions of the immune system for effective defence include:

1. Creation of barriers for the prevention of pathogens.
2. Identification of pathogens after their entry.
3. Elimination of pathogens.
4. Generation of immunological memory.
5. (Fig. **1**) depicts the immune system process and defense mechanism by means of a flowchart.

Creation of Barriers for the Prevention of Pathogens

The natural or first-line defence of our immune system are the natural barriers, which prevent the entry of pathogens from external environment, into our body. These natural barriers include physical barriers, chemical barriers, or biological barriers. Physical barriers include skin, mucosal layer of gastrointestinal tract, mucosal layer of genitourinary tract and mucosal layer of respiratory tract. Chemical barriers include the acidic pH of stomach, which destroys the pathogen before reaching its target site through the bloodstream. Besides this, sweat, saliva, mucus and tears also act as chemical barriers in the immune system, as they contain lysozyme, which destroys the pathogen, thereby preventing its entry into our body. Biological barriers to the immune system include common organisms on the skin and gut, which are harmless and use up food and space so that pathogenic bacteria do not have a chance to colonize themselves. Other than this, secretions like IgA (immunoglobulins) also act as an important biological barrier to immunity [6].

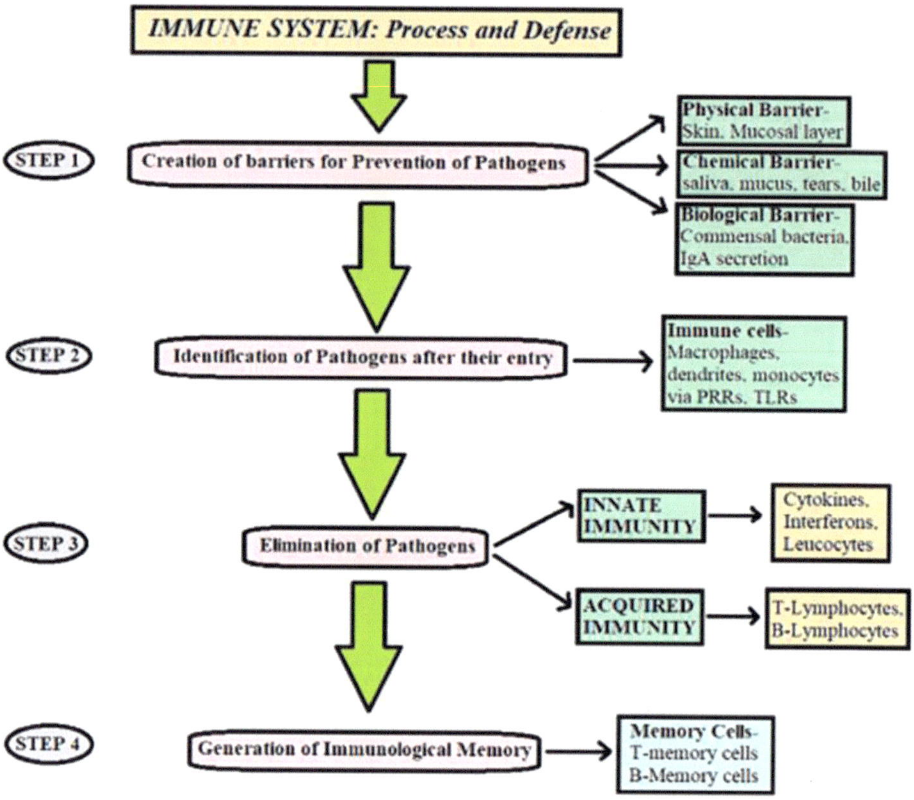

Fig. (1). Flowchart representing Immune system process and defense mechanism.

Identification of Pathogens After their Entry

Immune cells like macrophages, dendrites and monocytes of the innate immunity system are responsible for the recognition or identification of pathogens upon their entry. The recognition process depends upon pattern recognition receptors (PRRs), present on the immune cell's surface, which identify the molecular structure of the pathogen. This molecular structure is broadly similar to most kinds of pathogens and is termed microbe-associated molecular patterns (MAMPs) or pathogen-associated molecular patterns (PAMPs). The pattern recognition receptors consist of different toll-like receptors (TLRs), each of which is responsible for the identification of different pathogens like bacteria, viruses, fungi, and other parasites. Viruses are particularly identified by intracellular

TLRs. TLR-7 and TLR-8 found in immune cells are found to be important in the recognition of single-stranded RNA of coronavirus [7]. Viral genome type is detected *via* TLRs, which on identification, leads to interferon-mediated responses accordingly. TLR-3 is responsible for the detection of dsRNA, while TLR-7 and TLR-8 are responsible for the identification of ssRNA [8, 9].

Elimination of Pathogens

Once the pattern recognition receptors on immune cells recognize the pathogen, the defence mechanism of our body becomes active. First innate immunity is activated, and cytokines and interferons come into action. They signal cells to start cleaving RNA and reduce protein synthesis. Besides, nearby cells undergo apoptosis, thus causing inflammation. Interleukins, a type of cytokine, signal leucocytes to act and connect innate and acquired immune responses. Pathogens have antigens on their cell surface, which are recognized by T-lymphocytes, and they start proliferating and producing interleukins and interferons, which trigger the production of antigen-specific antibodies by B-lymphocytes. These antibodies neutralize or engulf the pathogen, thus enhancing the rate of phagocytosis [10]. Type-1 interferon (IFN-1) is expressed only after activation of PRR. IFN-1 contains thirteen IFN-α variants and one IFN-β in human beings, and these are secreted by hematopoietic cells and are responsible for action against ssRNA (present in SARS-CoV-19 virus), dsRNA and cytosolic DNA of viruses. Type-2 interferon (IFN-2) contains IFN-γ variants which, on pathogenic identification, start expression of IFN-stimulated genes (ISGs), which act by restricted replication of viral genomes by reduced protein synthesis [11].

Viral infections promote the release of interferon-alpha and interferon-beta, thereby inducing antiviral resistance by activation of natural killer cells. Virally infected cells are generally killed by natural killer cells, while the PRRs help in the maturation of dendritic cells for memorizing the viral processing and presentation for acquired immunity. Presentation of virally infected cells with MHC I antigens, present in respiratory epithelial cells, leads to activation of the $CD8^+$ receptor of T-lymphocytes, which directs the cell to release perforin for cell destruction by this pore-forming protein, while virally infected cells with MHC II antigen leads to activation of $CD4^+$ receptor of T-lymphocytes, which produces interleukin-2 and interferon-gamma for differentiation of B-lymphocytes, which in turn produce antiviral antibodies [12, 13]. Thus, T-lymphocytes activate cellular immunity, while B-lymphocytes activate humoral immunity.

Generation of Immunological Memory

Immunological memory is developed over some time. It is defined as the ability of the immune system to specifically recognize the antigen of a pathogen, previously encountered by the body, and initiate a suitable immune response against it. There are two types of immunological memories, one which is active at all times for months to years and the other which becomes passive after antigen encounter but becomes active whenever required. The first type of immune memory involves the persistent circulation of antibodies in the bloodstream, ranging from months to years, and prevents any such type of reinfection [14]. The second type of immune response involves retraction of antibodies, once the infection is over, but memory T-cells and B-cells for that function persist in our body in a passive state and become active as soon as the same pathogen is encountered by the body again. These memory cells have a long life of decades. This immunological memory forms the basis of vaccines for different diseases, including coronavirus [15, 16].

STRUCTURE OF SARS-COV-2

COVID-19 virus/coronavirus are spherical viruses with an average diameter of 60-150 nm. They possess a large molecular weight of approx. 35,000-40,000 kDa. They are enclosed in a multilayer protein envelope. The outer viral envelope is a lipid bilayer majorly composed of membrane protein, envelope protein and spike glycoprotein. The spike proteins are majorly responsible for the interaction of the virus with the host cell receptors [17]. The membrane proteins are the basic structural proteins that provide shape and protection to the virus. These membrane proteins play a major role during the developmental and pathogenesis stages of the life-cycle of the virus [18]. The envelope proteins are the minor structural proteins that protect the virus during the budding or morphogenetic developmental stage. Besides, these proteins also form ion channels in the lipid bilayer [19]. Besides these, three major proteins, coronaviruses of subgenus *Embecovirus*, possess Hemagglutinin esterase (HE) spike proteins which are homodimer transmembrane proteins and are responsible for attachment of the virus to host cell and destruction of the sialic acid membrane of host cells. These proteins are derived from hemagglutinin esterase fusion (HEF) proteins which are resistant to high temperature and low pH conditions, thereby forming a major source of virulence. The structure of the SARS-COV-2 virus is laid-out in (Fig. **2**) [20, 21].

The spike protein or S protein of the viral molecule is composed of two subdomains: S1 and S2 subdomains. S1 subdomain forms the head of the spike protein, while the S2 subdomain forms the stem part embedded in the viral envelope [22]. The S1 subdomain or head part consists of the receptor-binding domain, which attaches to the host cell, and the S2 subdomain or stem part contains protease enzyme, which on activation, helps infusion of the virus with host cell through receptor binding complex formation [23, 24]. After this fusion, the ion channels formed by envelope proteins help in the transference of the viral genome into the host cell. The viral genome of the COVID-19 virus is single-stranded positive-sense RNA (+ss RNA) [25]. Non-structural protein 1 (Nsp1) are responsible for processing and replication of the viral genome, and non-structural protein 2 (Nsp2) is responsible for modulation of the survival signalling pathway of the virus in the host cell [26]. Thus, in this way, the virus replicates and takes control of the host cell.

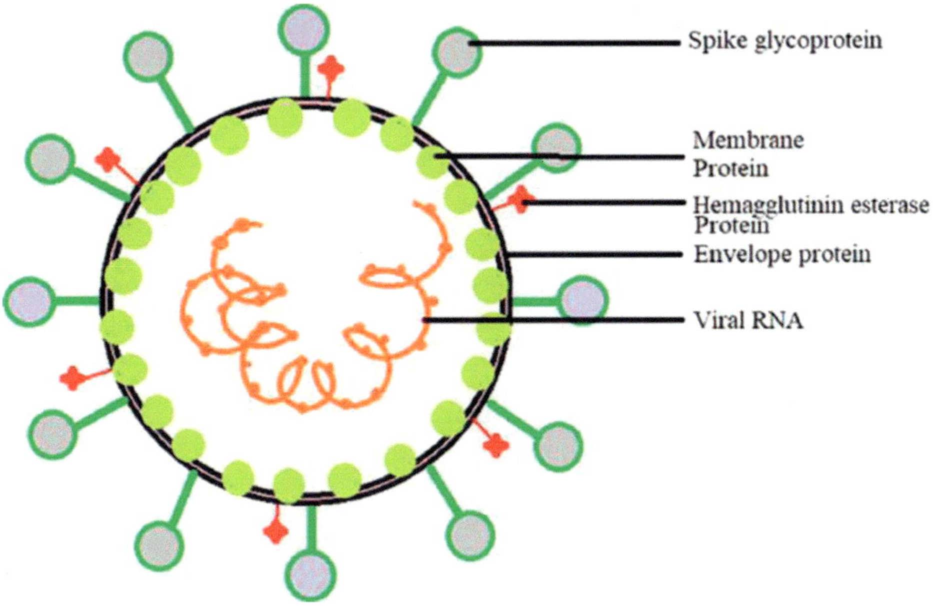

Fig. (2). Structure of SARS-CoV-2 virus.

Immunopathogenesis of COVID-19

For the COVID-19 pathogen, SARS-CoV-2, the "S-protein" present on the cell surface is involved in receptor recognition, attachment of virus, and its entrance into the host cell. Thus, this protein is an important component for the treatment research of coronavirus [27]. The "S-protein" of COVID-19 binds to angiotensin-converting enzyme-2 (ACE2) receptors found in the oral and nasal mucosa, lungs, gut, stomach, heart, and kidney. The enzyme is responsible for lowering blood pressure by catalysis of hydrolysis of angiotensin-II to angiotensin [28].

The disease shows different manifestations for different age groups as well as people with different morbidities. Healthy people with strong immunity suffer less, while elderly people with compromised immunity are at major risk [29]. Immunocompromised or old age people suffer from severe manifestations ranging from lymphopenia to multiple organ failure, while young people or the pediatric age group were found to be mostly asymptomatic cases and did not suffer much from the disease. Thus, this factor backs up the fact that immunity plays an important role in the pathogenesis of COVID-19 [30].

Viruses cause cell destruction in two different ways: one through cell pathogenic of the virus, which is a direct lysing effect, and the other through immune-response mediated destruction. Coronavirus causes cell death through immune-response mediated destruction, which is severe in the case of elderly people and less vigorous in the case of children and youngsters, thus making them asymptomatic carriers [31, 32]. The immunopathogenesis of the coronavirus is split into two stages: Non-severe and Severe Stages.

Non-Severe Stages

When a virus enters the host cell through the air pathway and rapidly multiplies inside the host to reach its alveoli, people with strong immunity respond timely with their cellular and humoral immune response, thereby, curbing the viral load reaching the alveoli and leading to recovery within 2-3 weeks. Humoral immunity checks the entry of the virus into new cells, thus, preventing new cells from being infected, while cellular immunity is actively involved in the destruction of infected cells. Thus, a strong immune system is an important requirement for the prevention of the severity of coronavirus [33, 34].

Severe Stage

Once the virus enters the host cell, it multiplies and reaches the lower tracheal region and alveoli. If the infection is not checked at this stage, the virus enters the systemic circulation and binds to ACE2 receptors present in the heart, liver, kidney, stomach, and other organs. Cellular immunity shows vigorous immune-response at this stage, producing cytokines like interferon-alpha, interferon-gamma, interleukin-1B, interleukin-6, interleukin-12, interleukin-18, interleukin-33, *etc*. and chemokines like CCL2, CCl3, CCL5, CXCL8, CXCL9, CXCL10, *etc*. This causes a condition known as "Cytokine storm", which is a severe immune response causing inflammation and damage to the organs of the host. This causes an increased risk of the thromboembolic phenomenon as well [35, 36].

NUTRITION AND IMMUNITY

The activation of immune response leads to the production of immunoglobulins, prostaglandins, chemokines, cytokines, leukotrienes, acute phase proteins and others, and for the production of these substances, the availability of substrates like amino acids, fatty acids and other nutritional sources is a must. Thus, nutrition and immunity are directly related to each other [37]. Besides, with increasing immune cells, following the response, a larger amount of DNA, RNA, proteins and lipids are required, and their biosynthesis is also dependent on amino acids, lipids, vitamins and other micronutrients. Thus, immunity is also indirectly dependent on nutrition [38].

The energy for metabolic activities requires various vitamins and minerals as cofactors. Amino acids are precursors for nucleic acids required for the functioning of immune cells and memory cells. Micronutrients like zinc, selenium, iron, magnesium, and folate are also important requisites for nucleotide synthesis information and other metabolic machinery controllers [39]. Vitamins such as vitamin A and vitamin D play a major role in gene expression in different cells and are important propagators of the maturation and differentiation of cells. Vitamin C and E also play an important role in the synthesis of various antioxidant enzymes which catalyse the immune response. Thus, nutrition lends a helping hand for a smooth and strong immune response [40].

Though all vitamins and micronutrients are important for the immunity of our body, vitamins A, C and D play an important role in immunity against COVID-19. Besides, micronutrients like zinc and copper also have a pivotal role in immunity against COVID-19 [41]. Their roles in COVID-19 are summarized as follows:

Vitamin A and Immunity Efficiency

Vitamin A is an important requirement for the differentiation, maturation and functioning of immune cells. Thus, a deficiency of the same would lead to impaired immune responses and increased exposure to pathogens. Vitamin A regulates neutrophil maturation, $CD4^+$ T-lymphocyte maturation, dendritic cell maturation, $CD8^+$ T-lymphocyte proliferation and the functioning of natural killer cells. Thus, deficiency of vitamin A, in general, leads to reduced or loss of phagocytic activity and impaired immune responses [42].

In the case of immunity against COVID-19, vitamin A decreases the effect, mortality rate and morbidity due to pneumonia, which is one of the fatal associated effects of COVID-19. In research, vitamin A supplementation is useful in reducing the severity of pneumonia effects as well as enhancing the clinical response rate [43].

Vitamin C and Immunity Efficiency

Vitamin C is a very important nutrient in terms of immunity. It is required for the biosynthesis of several important prerequisite factors of immune cells, like collagen and amino acids. It plays a pivotal role in leucocyte migration to the infection site, pathogen phagocytosis, functioning of natural killer cells, functioning of T-lymphocytes and antibody production. Thus, deficiency in vitamin C content leads to impairment of T-lymphocyte-mediated immune response as well as immune memory [44, 45].

In terms of immunity against COVID-19, vitamin C is an important source to fight against respiratory diseases and is often given as a precautionary measure against COVID-19. In research, vitamin C was found to decrease the incidence of pneumonia, the severity of pneumonia as well as the duration of pneumonia. The vitamin was also found to be useful in case of preventing common cold and upper respiratory tract infections. Since pneumonia is an important associated mortality factor for COVID-19, therefore vitamin C plays an important role in counteracting or preventing COVID-19 by providing stronger immune responses [46].

Vitamin D and Immunity Efficiency

Vitamin D receptors are present in a majority of immune cells, and some of them are even synthesizing 1,25-dihydroxyvitamin D_3, the active form of vitamin D from its precursor; thus, the importance of vitamin D in the immune system can be estimated through this [47]. Vitamin D progresses the differentiation of monocytes to macrophages, increases phagocytosis of infected cells, production of superoxide, thereby enhancing innate immunity. It helps the memory cells in recognizing antigens and triggering the body system to generate a corresponding immune response. Vitamin D also helps in controlling the proliferation of T-lymphocytes thereby, helping in controlling the "cytokine storm" in severe cases [48].

In terms of immunity against COVID-19, vitamin D shares a linear inverse relationship with respiratory tract infection, implying that as the percentage of vitamin D decreases in the body, the susceptibility to respiratory tract infections increases [49]. In research, patients with respiratory tract infections presented great improvement on being supplemented with vitamin D. Vitamin D was found to play a pivotal role in decreasing acute respiratory tract infections, and its decreased percentage was found to be a helping hand for the development of pneumonia-like infection [50].

Zinc Micronutrient and Immunity Efficiency

Zinc is an important micronutrient for the immune system. It helps in regulating the number of T- and B- lymphocytes, and its deficiency was found to cause a severe dip in the number of immune cells, thus affecting immunity of the body.

Zinc is important for macrophagic phagocytosis and function against natural killer cells; thus, zinc deficiency also affects innate immunity. At times, zinc chelation and zinc malabsorption were also found to have marked effects on immune responses and antiviral activity of the body [51].

In terms of immunity against COVID-19, zinc plays a very important role in the destruction of coronavirus, thus, having a direct effect on COVID-19. Zinc is found to inhibit RNA polymerase, which is an important constituent required for the replication of RNA viruses, like coronavirus. Once the replication of coronavirus is checked in time, the infection can automatically be curbed. Thus, zinc is assumed to have *in vitro* inhibitory effects on coronavirus. Thus, zinc plays a major supplementary role in curbing coronavirus [52].

Copper Micronutrient and Immunity Efficiency

Copper promotes the functioning of neutrophils, macrophages and monocytes and natural killer cells, thus playing an important role in innate immunity. It also promotes T-lymphocyte responses and interleukin production. Copper deficiency is associated with susceptibility to pathogenic infections. Copper deficiency also increases susceptibility towards diarrhoea and pneumonia and recurrent respiratory tract infection. So, copper is an important micronutrient in the treatment of respiratory infections, therefore is considered to be an important nutrient for immunity against COVID-19 [53, 54].

Thus, in this way, various micronutrients act as immunity boosters against COVID-19.

HERD IMMUNITY AND CORONAVIRUS

Herd immunity is a type of indirect prevention of the spread of infection. Herd immunity has proved its worth in controlling the cases of coronavirus, in places like slums or ghettos, or even villages, especially in developing or underprivileged countries [55]. Herd immunity is a kind of indirect immunity, where the number of vaccinated or immune people and healthy or uninfected people supersede the number of infected people by a large difference, thereby preventing or reducing the rate of person-to-person transmission of a highly communicable disease like COVID-19. Thus, in this way, herd immunity can act as a check to the spread of COVID-19 [56].

NATURAL PRODUCTS AND IMMUNITY AGAINST COVID-19

During the COVID-19 pandemic, many natural products from plants and herbs were found to be extremely helpful in the prevention and treatment of the disease.

Some major plant products taken as natural medicines include tulsi (*Ocimum sanctum*), giloy (*Tinospora cardifolia*), ashwagandha (*Withania somnifera*), dalchini (*Cinnamomum Verum*), sunthi (*Zingiber officinale*) and Marich (*Piper nigrum*). They acted as immunity boosters and helped in the prevention and even reduction of the severity of corona infection. These plants contained several bioactive chemical compounds which proved helpful in boosting immunity by providing precursors for bioactivation and production of immune cells [57]. The chemical composition and role of these plants in immunity against COVID-19 can be summarized as follows:

Tulsi as Immunity Booster

Tulsi plant (*Ocimum*) possesses certain bioactive compounds like eugenol, phenols and linoleic acid, and therefore it shows a variety of biological activities as well, and acts as antimicrobial, antidiarrheal, antipyretic, analgesic, hepato-protective, reno-protective, cardio-protective, antiviral, anti-inflammatory and antioxidant. Due to its anti-inflammatory and antioxidant properties, Tulsi protects the cells from any chemically induced injury and also protects them from oxidative injury, by periodical clearing of free radicals from the body [58].

Tulsi boosts the defence mechanism of the body against COVID-19. Chemical constituents like carnosol, rosmarinic acid, apigenin, ursolic acid and circilineol, present in tulsi augment SRBC (sheep blood red cells) agglutinins titres and decrease cyclo-oxygenase-2 and lipo-oxygenase-2 [59]. Besides, it causes upregulation of interleukin-2, interferon-gamma and tumour necrosis factor-alpha and downregulation of interleukin-1beta. It also produces specific antibodies which help the body in T-cell-dependent immune responses. Thus, these activities and properties represent the vital role of the tulsi plant in enhancing immunity against COVID-19 [60].

Giloy as Immunity Booster

Giloy also acts as an important immunity enhancer and therefore, has been approved by Food and drug administration (FDA) as a remedial medication in COVID-19. *Tinospora* possesses great antiviral, anti-inflammatory, anti-analgesic, antipyretic, anti-fungal, anti-diabetic and antioxidant activities. Due to its antioxidant properties, it detoxifies the body at a great pace and helps in building better immunity. The plant contains chemical constituents like alkaloids, terpenoids, lignans and steroids that have a great impact on the pharmacological properties of the plant in treating various diseases [61]. The stem of giloy is found to have major antipyretic and antioxidant activities and the juice of stem was found helpful in preventing as well as treating COVID-19 symptoms. The phytochemicals like tinosporine, tinosporaside, cordifol, heptacosanol, clerodane, berberine and magniflorine present in the stem of *Tinospora,* have proved beneficial in treating respiratory tract infections, common cough and cold and high fever. Besides, these phytoconstituents also help in the biosynthesis and repairment of immune cells, thereby, boosting the immunity of the body against COVID-19 [62].

Ashwagandha as Immunity Booster

Ashwagandha or *Withania somnifera* have proved their worth during COVID times, as a faster recovery agent for sufferers of coronavirus. Owing to its great success as a medicine in COVID-19, recently ministry of Ayush, India and the London School of Hygiene and tropical medicine, U.K. have collaborated to investigate and conduct clinical trials for the same. Ashwagandha possesses immunomodulatory, anti-inflammatory and antioxidant properties. Phytoconstituents like somniferine, withamine, somnine, and withanaminine alkaloids from the root extract of the plant are important factors for curbing respiratory infections, acting as an anti-inflammatory agent and acting as stress reducer agents. Besides, hygrine, hentriacotane, mesoanaferine and visamine present in the methanolic extract of plant stem are also responsible for boosting immunity and rejuvenating cells. It also possesses certain amino acids, which are precursors for the biosynthesis of the nucleic acid of important immune cells [62].

Dalchini as Immunity Booster

Dalchini or *Cinnamomum* has been an important immunity booster since ancient times. The stem bark of the plant is majorly responsible for its immunity enhancing properties. It contains important phytoconstituents like cinnamaldehyde, benzaldehyde, cuminaldehyde and terpenes, which are responsible for the increased phagocytic index, serum immunoglobulin levels and decreased reduction in neutrophil count. The studies reveal that high doses of cinnamon have enhanced effects on cellular as well as humoral immunity. Cinnamaldehyde present in dalchini acts as a strong regulator of monocyte or macrophage-mediated immunity. It is also responsible for enhanced rates of co-stimulatory molecule production for immune cells and also for enhanced activity of the pattern recognition system. Cinnamaldehyde and cinnamophilin present in dalchini act as an anticoagulative and anti-atherosclerotic agent and thus prevent clumping of platelets and blood corpuscles, therefore was found to be an important agent for the treatment of COVID symptoms and for decreasing CRP (C-reactive protein) values [63].

Sunthi as Immunity Booster

Sunthi, ginger, or *Zingiber officinale* is also a good immunity booster and enhances both cellular and humoral immunity. The phytoconstituents present in the plant include nevirapine, beta-sitosterol, 6-gingediol, germacrene, methyl---shogaol, linalool and zingiberene are found to inhibit viral replication [64]. Beta-sitosterol is, in fact, the most potent inhibitor of reverse transcriptase enzyme and is considered to be one of the major antiviral components. Thus, the rhizome of the plant is useful in treating the COVID-19 virus, as well. Besides, gingerols and shogaols inhibit the synthesis of interleukin-1 and 8, without any modulation in IL-6 levels, indicating enhancement of immunity [65, 66].

Marich as Immunity Booster

Marich or *Piper nigrum* acts as an indirect agent for immunity boosting. It enhances the bioavailability of drugs and thus acts as a supplement and support for increasing the therapeutic effect of drugs or vaccines. The plant possesses antihypertensive, antipyretic, antioxidant, antispasmodic and antihemorrhagic agents. Its phytoconstituents include piperine which maintains the balance of cytokine production and reduces the accumulation of inflammatory cells. It also serves to increase the rate of activation of T and B cell proliferation, thus enhancing cellular as well as humoral immunity [67].

VACCINATION AND IMMUNITY AGAINST COVID-19

Various vaccines have been developed by different countries for immunity against COVID-19. Vaccines boost the immunological memory of the immune system, thereby preventing the occurrence of disease. Vaccines safely deliver the COVID immunogen into the body, to train the immune system to recognize the viral pathogen and trigger an immediate acquired immune response, when a coronavirus attacks the body. The immunogen could be an attenuated coronavirus, protein capsid of virus, safe vector of virus or RNA or DNA of the virus. Based on these immunogens, four types of vaccines have been developed by different countries. The four types include inactivated or weakened vaccines, protein-based vaccines, viral vector vaccines and RNA and DNA vaccines [68, 69]. Thus, vaccines are a source that helps in developing the memory of our immune systems. They develop passive immunity against COVID-19 in our bodies, so that next when they encounter the active form of the same virus, they can immediately remember the PRR and take immediate action to weaken or subdue the virus. So basically, vaccines are proving to be immunity boosters against the SARS-CoV-2 virus by acting as a weaker pre-exposure to the enemy attack.

Different approved vaccines, produced by different countries include Moderna (RNA vaccine) from the United States of America, AstraZeneca (viral vector vaccine) from the United Kingdom, Pfizer/BioNtech (RNA vaccine) from Germany, Sinovac (inactivated vaccine) from China, Covishield (inactivated vaccine) from India, and Johnson & Johnson/Jannsen (viral vector vaccine) from the United States of America.

Moderna vaccines are prevalent as a two-dose vaccine for people above 18 years of age. A booster dose of the same has been introduced recently, taken after the completion of five months of the second dose. The vaccine has also been approved for "mix and matches" booster dose after the completion of two primary dosages. The common side effects of this vaccine include tiredness, headache, joint inflammation, swollen lymph nodes, muscular pain, nausea, fever and vomiting [70].

AstraZeneca vaccine (Vaxzevria) is recommended for a dosage of two doses to be taken at an interval of 8-12 weeks in the dosage limit of 0.5ml each. AstraZeneca vaccines also support the usage of heterologous doses. Common side-effects of vaccine doses include tiredness, headache, fever and pain [71].

Pfizer vaccine recommends a dose cycle of two shots at an interval of 21 days. Older and immunocompromised people are suggested to receive an additional primary dose after 28 days-5 months of the second dose. The recommended age for this vaccine is above five years. Common side effects include fever, nausea, dizziness and body ache. People with an allergy to polyethene glycols should avoid these doses as they can express severe allergic reactions [72].

Covaxin is an indigenous Indian vaccine produced by Bharat Biotech. WHO has recommended the usage of vaccines with a two-dose cycle, to be administered at an interval of 4 weeks. WHO also recommends a provision for an additional dose of the vaccine to immunocompromised and elderly people. Heterologous usage of doses for the vaccine is also under trails [73].

CONCLUSION

Thus, it can be concluded that immunity plays a pivotal role in the prevention and treatment of COVID-19. Stronger immunity means lesser suffering or complete prevention from COVID-19. Immunity is based on factors like age, physical fitness, and some pre-existing diseases. Immunity can be boosted by several health supplements like vitamins and micronutrients. Immunity was found to have a direct impact on the immunopathogenesis of the process of corona disease. Various plant products were also found quite effective in enhancing the immune response system of the body. Daily dosage of such natural products has shown effective results in boosting immunity gradually, without any side effects. Besides, vaccination has also been proven as the last resort to provide acquired immunity, which is an effective measure against COVID-19. So, to conclude, it can be rightly said that immunity has a very important role in our fight against the existing pandemic, COVID-19.

CONSENT FOR PUBLICATION

Not applicable.

CONFLICT OF INTEREST

The authors declare no conflict of interest, financial or otherwise.

ACKNOWLEDGEMENTS

The author wants to thank Dr. Tahmeena Khan and Dr. Alfred Lawrence for their insightful reviews in preparing this chapter.

REFERENCES

[1] Calder PC. Feeding the immune system. Proc Nutr Soc 2013; 72(3): 299-309. [http://dx.doi.org/10.1017/S0029665113001286] [PMID: 23688939]

[2] Gombart AF, Pierre A, Maggini S. A review of micronutrients and the immune system–working in harmony to reduce the risk of infection. Nutrients 2020; 12(1): 236. [http://dx.doi.org/10.3390/nu12010236] [PMID: 31963293]

[3] Leung C. Clinical features of deaths in the novel coronavirus epidemic in China. Rev Med Virol 2020; 30(3): e2103. [http://dx.doi.org/10.1002/rmv.2103] [PMID: 32175637]

[4] Wu D, Wu T, Liu Q, Yang Z. The SARS-CoV-2 outbreak: What we know. Int J Infect Dis 2020; 94: 44-8. [http://dx.doi.org/10.1016/j.ijid.2020.03.004] [PMID: 32171952]

[5] Dosch SF, Mahajan SD, Collins AR. SARS coronavirus spike protein-induced innate immune response occurs *via* activation of the NF-κB pathway in human monocyte macrophages *in vitro*. Virus Res 2009; 142(1-2): 19-27. [http://dx.doi.org/10.1016/j.virusres.2009.01.005] [PMID: 19185596]

[6] Hu W, Yen YT, Singh S, Kao CL, Wu-Hsieh BA. SARS-CoV regulates immune function-related gene expression in human monocytic cells. Viral Immunol 2012; 25(4): 277-88. [http://dx.doi.org/10.1089/vim.2011.0099] [PMID: 22876772]

[7] Wang Y, Liu L. The membrane protein of severe acute respiratory syndrome coronavirus functions as a novel cytosolic pathogen-associated molecular pattern to promote beta interferon induction *via* a Toll-like-receptor-related TRAF3-independent mechanism. MBio 2016; 7(1): e01872-15. [http://dx.doi.org/10.1128/mBio.01872-15] [PMID: 26861016]

[8] Nie L, Cai SY, Shao JZ, Chen J. Toll-like receptors, associated biological roles, and signaling networks in non-mammals. Front Immunol 2018; 9: 1523. [http://dx.doi.org/10.3389/fimmu.2018.01523] [PMID: 30034391]

[9] Kawasaki T, Kawai T. Toll-like receptor signaling pathways. Front Immunol 2014; 5: 461. [http://dx.doi.org/10.3389/fimmu.2014.00461] [PMID: 25309543]

[10] Al-Qahtani AA, Lyroni K, Aznaourova M, *et al.* Middle east respiratory syndrome corona virus spike glycoprotein suppresses macrophage responses *via* DPP4-mediated induction of IRAK-M and PPARγ. Oncotarget. 2017; 8 (6): 9053. [http://dx.doi.org/10.18632/oncotarget.14754]

[11] Kopitar-Jerala N. The role of interferons in inflammation and inflammasome activation. Front Immunol 2017; 8: 873. [http://dx.doi.org/10.3389/fimmu.2017.00873] [PMID: 28791024]

[12] García-Sastre A, Biron CA. Type 1 interferons and the virus-host relationship: a lesson in detente. Science. 2006; 312 (5775): 879-882. [http://dx.doi.org/10.1126/science.1125676]

[13] Sallard E, Lescure FX, Yazdanpanah Y, Mentre F, Peiffer-Smadja N. Type 1 interferons as a potential treatment against COVID-19. Antiviral Res 2020; 178: 104791. [http://dx.doi.org/10.1016/j.antiviral.2020.104791] [PMID: 32275914]

[14] Pawelec G, Larbi A, Derhovanessian E. Senescence of the human immune system. J Comp Pathol 2010; 142 (Suppl. 1): S39-44. [http://dx.doi.org/10.1016/j.jcpa.2009.09.005] [PMID: 19897208]

[15] Pera A, Campos C, López N, *et al.* Immunosenescence: Implications for response to infection and vaccination in older people. Maturitas 2015; 82(1): 50-5. [http://dx.doi.org/10.1016/j.maturitas.2015.05.004] [PMID: 26044074]

[16] Calder PC. Nutrition, immunity and COVID-19. BMJ Nutrition, Prevention & Health 2020; 3(1): 74-92. [http://dx.doi.org/10.1136/bmjnph-2020-000085] [PMID: 33230497]

[17] Lalchhandama K. The chronicles of coronaviruses: the electron microscope, the doughnut, and the spike. Sci Vis 2020; 20(2): 78-92. [http://dx.doi.org/10.33493/scivis.20.02.03]

[18] Timani KA, Ye L, Ye L, Zhu Y, Wu Z, Gong Z. Cloning, sequencing, expression, and purification of SARS-associated coronavirus nucleocapsid protein for serodiagnosis of SARS. J Clin Virol 2004; 30(4): 309-12. [http://dx.doi.org/10.1016/j.jcv.2004.01.001] [PMID: 15163419]

[19] Cao Y, Yang R, Lee I, *et al.* Characterization of the SARS-CoV-2 E Protein: Sequence, Structure, Viroporin, and Inhibitors. Protein Sci 2021; 30(6): 1114-30. [http://dx.doi.org/10.1002/pro.4075] [PMID: 33813796]

[20] Wang M, Ludwig K, Böttcher C, Veit M. The role of stearate attachment to the hemagglutinin-esterase-fusion glycoprotein HEF of influenza C virus. Cell Microbiol 2016; 18(5): 692-704. [http://dx.doi.org/10.1111/cmi.12541] [PMID: 26518983]

[21] Yu J, Hika B, Liu R, *et al.* The hemagglutinin-esterase fusion glycoprotein is a primary determinant of the exceptional thermal and acid stability of influenza D virus. MSphere 2017; 2(4): e00254-17. [http://dx.doi.org/10.1128/mSphere.00254-17] [PMID: 28808690]

[22] Wang MY, Zhao R, Gao LJ, Gao XF, Wang DP, Cao JM. SARS-CoV-2: structure, biology, and structure-based therapeutics development. Front Cell Infect Microbiol 2020; 10: 587269. [http://dx.doi.org/10.3389/fcimb.2020.587269] [PMID: 33324574]

[23] Lu R, Zhao X, Li J, *et al.* Genomic characterisation and epidemiology of 2019 novel coronavirus: implications for virus origins and receptor binding. Lancet 2020; 395(10224): 565-74. [http://dx.doi.org/10.1016/S0140-6736(20)30251-8] [PMID: 32007145]

[24] Brian DA, Baric RS. Coronavirus genome structure and replication 2005. [http://dx.doi.org/10.1007/3-540-26765-4_1]

[25] Gao Y, Yan L, Huang Y, *et al.* Structure of the RNA-dependent RNA polymerase from COVID-19

virus. Science 2020; 368(6492): 779-82.
[http://dx.doi.org/10.1126/science.abb7498] [PMID: 32277040]

[26] Naqvi AAT, Fatima K, Mohammad T, *et al.* Insights into SARS-CoV-2 genome, structure, evolution, pathogenesis and therapies: Structural genomics approach. Biochim Biophys Acta Mol Basis Dis 2020; 1866(10): 165878.
[http://dx.doi.org/10.1016/j.bbadis.2020.165878] [PMID: 32544429]

[27] Xu H, Zhong L, Deng J, *et al.* High expression of ACE2 receptor of 2019-nCoV on the epithelial cells of oral mucosa. Int J Oral Sci 2020; 12(1): 8.
[http://dx.doi.org/10.1038/s41368-020-0074-x] [PMID: 32094336]

[28] Donoghue M, Hsieh F, Baronas E, *et al.* A novel angiotensin-converting enzyme-related carboxypeptidase (ACE2) converts angiotensin I to angiotensin 1-9. Circ Res 2000; 87(5): E1-9.
[http://dx.doi.org/10.1161/01.RES.87.5.e1] [PMID: 10969042]

[29] Cruz AT, Zeichner SL. COVID-19 in children: initial characterization of the pediatric disease. Pediatrics 2020; 145(6): e20200834.
[http://dx.doi.org/10.1542/peds.2020-0834] [PMID: 32179659]

[30] Porter DD. Destruction of virus-infected cells by immunological mechanisms. Annu Rev Microbiol 1971; 25(1): 283-90.
[http://dx.doi.org/10.1146/annurev.mi.25.100171.001435] [PMID: 5005028]

[31] Shi Y, Wang Y, Shao C, *et al.* COVID-19 infection: the perspectives on immune responses. Cell Death Differ 2020; 27(5): 1451-4.
[http://dx.doi.org/10.1038/s41418-020-0530-3] [PMID: 32205856]

[32] Bonavia A, Zelus BD, Wentworth DE, Talbot PJ, Holmes KV. Identification of a receptor-binding domain of the spike glycoprotein of human coronavirus HCoV-229E. J Virol 2003; 77(4): 2530-8.
[http://dx.doi.org/10.1128/JVI.77.4.2530-2538.2003] [PMID: 12551991]

[33] Jin Y, Yang H, Ji W, *et al.* Virology, epidemiology, pathogenesis, and control of COVID-19. Viruses 2020; 12(4): 372.
[http://dx.doi.org/10.3390/v12040372] [PMID: 32230900]

[34] Widjaja G, Turki Jalil A, Sulaiman Rahman H, *et al.* Humoral immune mechanisms involved in protective and pathological immunity during COVID-19. Hum Immunol 2021; 82(10): 733-45.
[http://dx.doi.org/10.1016/j.humimm.2021.06.011] [PMID: 34229864]

[35] Cameron MJ, Bermejo-Martin JF, Danesh A, Muller MP, Kelvin DJ. Human immunopathogenesis of severe acute respiratory syndrome (SARS). Virus Res 2008; 133(1): 13-9.
[http://dx.doi.org/10.1016/j.virusres.2007.02.014] [PMID: 17374415]

[36] Cattaneo M, Bertinato EM, Birocchi S, *et al.* Pulmonary embolism or pulmonary thrombosis in COVID-19? Is the recommendation to use high-dose heparin for thromboprophylaxis justified? Thromb Haemost 2020; 120(8): 1230-2.
[http://dx.doi.org/10.1055/s-0040-1712097] [PMID: 32349132]

[37] Maggini S, Wintergerst ES, Beveridge S, Hornig DH. Selected vitamins and trace elements support immune function by strengthening epithelial barriers and cellular and humoral immune responses. Br J Nutr 2007; 98(S1) (Suppl. 1): S29-35.
[http://dx.doi.org/10.1017/S0007114507832971] [PMID: 17922955]

[38] Alpert PT. The role of vitamins and minerals on the immune system. Home Health Care Manage Pract 2017; 29(3): 199-202.
[http://dx.doi.org/10.1177/1084822317713300]

[39] Wu D, Lewis ED, Pae M, Meydani SN. Nutritional modulation of immune function: analysis of evidence, mechanisms, and clinical relevance. Front Immunol 2019; 9: 3160.
[http://dx.doi.org/10.3389/fimmu.2018.03160] [PMID: 30697214]

[40] Villamor E, Fawzi WW. Effects of vitamin a supplementation on immune responses and correlation

with clinical outcomes. Clin Microbiol Rev 2005; 18(3): 446-64.
[http://dx.doi.org/10.1128/CMR.18.3.446-464.2005] [PMID: 16020684]

[41] Ross AC. Vitamin A and retinoic acid in T cell–related immunity. Am J Clin Nutr 2012; 96(5): 1166S-72S.
[http://dx.doi.org/10.3945/ajcn.112.034637] [PMID: 23053562]

[42] Larange A, Cheroutre H. Retinoic acid and retinoic acid receptors as pleiotropic modulators of the immune system. Annu Rev Immunol 2016; 34(1): 369-94.
[http://dx.doi.org/10.1146/annurev-immunol-041015-055427] [PMID: 27168242]

[43] Oliveira LM, Teixeira FME, Sato MN. Impact of retinoic acid on immune cells and inflammatory diseases. Mediators Inflamm 2018; 2018: 1-17.
[http://dx.doi.org/10.1155/2018/3067126] [PMID: 30158832]

[44] Carr A, Maggini S. Vitamin C and immune function. Nutrients 2017; 9(11): 1211.
[http://dx.doi.org/10.3390/nu9111211] [PMID: 29099763]

[45] Hemilä H. Vitamin C and infections. Nutrients 2017; 9(4): 339.
[http://dx.doi.org/10.3390/nu9040339] [PMID: 28353648]

[46] Jacob RA, Kelley DS, Pianalto FS, *et al.* Immunocompetence and oxidant defense during ascorbate depletion of healthy men. Am J Clin Nutr 1991; 54(6) (Suppl.): 1302S-9S.
[http://dx.doi.org/10.1093/ajcn/54.6.1302s] [PMID: 1962587]

[47] Di Rosa M, Malaguarnera M, Nicoletti F, Malaguarnera L. Vitamin D3: a helpful immuno-modulator. Immunology 2011; 134(2): 123-39.
[http://dx.doi.org/10.1111/j.1365-2567.2011.03482.x] [PMID: 21896008]

[48] Sassi F, Tamone C, D'Amelio P. Vitamin D: nutrient, hormone, and immunomodulator. Nutrients 2018; 10(11): 1656.
[http://dx.doi.org/10.3390/nu10111656] [PMID: 30400332]

[49] Medrano M, Carrillo-Cruz E, Montero I, Perez-Simon J. Vitamin D: effect on haematopoiesis and immune system and clinical applications. Int J Mol Sci 2018; 19(9): 2663.
[http://dx.doi.org/10.3390/ijms19092663] [PMID: 30205552]

[50] Prietl B, Treiber G, Pieber T, Amrein K. Vitamin D and immune function. Nutrients 2013; 5(7): 2502-21.
[http://dx.doi.org/10.3390/nu5072502] [PMID: 23857223]

[51] Bonaventura P, Benedetti G, Albarède F, Miossec P. Zinc and its role in immunity and inflammation. Autoimmun Rev 2015; 14(4): 277-85.
[http://dx.doi.org/10.1016/j.autrev.2014.11.008] [PMID: 25462582]

[52] Read SA, Obeid S, Ahlenstiel C, Ahlenstiel G. The role of zinc in antiviral immunity. Adv Nutr 2019; 10(4): 696-710.
[http://dx.doi.org/10.1093/advances/nmz013] [PMID: 31305906]

[53] te Velthuis AJW, van den Worm SHE, Sims AC, Baric RS, Snijder EJ, van Hemert MJ. Zn(2+) inhibits coronavirus and arterivirus RNA polymerase activity *in vitro* and zinc ionophores block the replication of these viruses in cell culture. PLoS Pathog 2010; 6(11): e1001176.
[http://dx.doi.org/10.1371/journal.ppat.1001176] [PMID: 21079686]

[54] Singh N, Satpute S, Polkam N, *et al.* Design, synthesis and evaluation of 4H-Chromene-4-one analogues as potential Anti-bacterial and Anti-fungal agents. Chem Biol Lett 2020; 7(1): 27-40.

[55] Randolph HE, Barreiro LB. Herd Immunity: Understanding COVID-19. Immunity 2020; 52(5): 737-41.
[http://dx.doi.org/10.1016/j.immuni.2020.04.012] [PMID: 32433946]

[56] Metcalf CJE, Ferrari M, Graham AL, Grenfell BT. Understanding herd immunity. Trends Immunol 2015; 36(12): 753-5.

[http://dx.doi.org/10.1016/j.it.2015.10.004] [PMID: 26683689]

[57] Hemalatha R, Babu KN, Karthik M, Ramesh R, Kumar BD, Kumar PU. Immunomodulatory activity and Th1/Th2 cytokine response of Ocimum sanctum in myelosuppressed swiss albino mice. Trends in Medical Research 2011; 6(1): 23-31. [http://dx.doi.org/10.3923/tmr.2011.23.31]

[58] Gautam MK, Goel RK. Toxicological study of Ocimum sanctum Linn leaves: hematological, biochemical, and histopathological studies. J Toxicol 2014; 2014: 1-9. [http://dx.doi.org/10.1155/2014/135654] [PMID: 24616736]

[59] Singh N, Pandey J. DABCO catalyzed, green and efficient, one-pot multicomponent synthesis of 5-aminopyrazole-4-carbonitrile. Curr Res Green Sustainable Chem 2021; 4: 100134. [http://dx.doi.org/10.1016/j.crgsc.2021.100134]

[60] Jamshidi N, Cohen MM. The clinical efficacy and safety of Tulsi in humans: a systematic review of the literature. Evid Based Complement Alternat Med 2017; 2017: 1-13. [http://dx.doi.org/10.1155/2017/9217567] [PMID: 28400848]

[61] Singh N, Pandey J. One-pot, water-mediated, H_2O_2-HCl catalysed synthesis of Benzazepines. Asian J Chem 2020; 32(5): 1165-8. [http://dx.doi.org/10.14233/ajchem.2020.22574]

[62] Singh N, Bhalla M, De Jager P, Gilca M. An overview on ashwagandha: a Rasayana (rejuvenator) of Ayurveda. Afr J Tradit Complement Altern Med 2011; 8(5S) (Suppl.): 208-13. [http://dx.doi.org/10.4314/ajtcam.v8i5S.9] [PMID: 22754076]

[63] Lee BJ, Kim YJ, Cho DH, Sohn NW, Kang H. Immunomodulatory effect of water extract of cinnamon on anti-CD3-induced cytokine responses and p38, JNK, ERK1/2, and STAT4 activation. Immunopharmacol Immunotoxicol 2011; 33(4): 714-22. [http://dx.doi.org/10.3109/08923973.2011.564185] [PMID: 22053946]

[64] Singh N, Pandey J. Advances in Henry Reaction: A Versatile Method in Organic Synthesis. Mini Rev Org Chem 2020; 17(3): 297-308. [http://dx.doi.org/10.2174/1570193X16666190214150144]

[65] Habib SHM, Makpol S, Hamid NAA, Das S, Ngah WZW, Yusof YAM. Ginger extract (Zingiber officinale) has anti-cancer and anti-inflammatory effects on ethionine-induced hepatoma rats. Clinics (São Paulo) 2008; 63(6): 807-13. [http://dx.doi.org/10.1590/S1807-59322008000600017] [PMID: 19061005]

[66] Zehsaz F, Farhangi N, Mirheidari L. Clinical immunology The effect of Zingiber officinale R. rhizomes (ginger) on plasma pro-inflammatory cytokine levels in well-trained male endurance runners. Cent Eur J Immunol 2014; 2(2): 174-80. [http://dx.doi.org/10.5114/ceji.2014.43719] [PMID: 26155120]

[67] Srivastava AK, Singh VK. Biological action of Piper nigrum-the king of spices. Eur J Biol Res 2017; 7(3): 223-33. [http://dx.doi.org/10.5281/zenodo.839039]

[68] Callaway E. COVID vaccine excitement builds as Moderna reports third positive result. Nature 2020, 587(7834): 337-8. [http://dx.doi.org/10.1038/d41586-020-03248-7] [PMID: 33199901]

[69] Liu C, Zhou Q, Li Y, *et al.* Research and development on therapeutic agents and vaccines for COVID-19 and related human coronavirus diseases. ACS Cent Sci 2020; 6(3): 315-31. [http://dx.doi.org/10.1021/acscentsci.0c00272] [PMID: 32226821]

[70] Mallapaty S, Callaway E. What scientists do and don't know about the Oxford-AstraZeneca COVID vaccine. Nature 2021; 592(7852): 15-27. [http://dx.doi.org/10.1038/d41586-021-00785-7]

[71] Food and Drug Administration (US). FDA shortens interval for booster dose of Moderna COVID-19

Vaccine to five months. Moderna COVID-19 Vaccine 2022.

[72] World Health Organization (WHO). The Oxford/Astrazeneca COVID-19 vaccine:what you need to know. 2021.

[73] Centre for Disease control and Prevention (US). Pfizer-BioNTech. General information 2022.

[74] World Health Organization (WHO). The Bharat Biotech BBV152 COVAXIN vaccine against COVID-19: what you need to know 2021.

SUBJECT INDEX

A

B

C

Tahmeena Khan & Alfred J. Lawrence (Eds.)

D

E

F

G

H

I

W

X

Z

Made in the USA
Las Vegas, NV
04 November 2026

57431856R00109